Supercharging Your Weight-loss Meal

The healthy smoothie way

Content

Introduction

For a large number of us it might be hard to expend the suggested day by day measures of organic products in vegetables; anyway, a tall glass of smoothie for breakfast or a titbit can assist us with meeting our everyday necessities.

While numerous individuals drink smoothies as a supper substitute to help with weight reduction, a genuine advantage of smoothies is in the nutrients and supplements that originate from the solid fixings that are mixed up.

Smoothies are an incredible method to expend vegetables in their crude and most nutritious structure, and not at all like squeezing, the fibre substance of the fixings in the smoothie is held, bringing about a more advantageous and all the more fulfilling drink.

Have a go at utilizing a rainbow of brilliant foods grown from the ground to incorporate a wide scope of cell reinforcements that can help battle numerous sicknesses including malignant growth and coronary illness. Use smoothies as an approach to expend vegetables that you and your family may not eat something else.

You will be amazed at how well the flavour of numerous vegetables can be veiled by the flavour and pleasantness from the natural products that you blend in.

Freeze natural products, for example, berries, mangoes, and peaches when they are in season and drop the solidified organic products into the blender for a delightful solidified beverage that you can appreciate all year. Add ice to make a slushie-like smoothie, or yogurt to give it a milkshake consistency. In this segment you will discover plans, for example, Banana and Mango Smoothie. In any case, the best smoothies are those that are modified to your taste and healthful needs.

Get imaginative and include fixings, for example, Greek yogurt, a sprinkle of organic product squeeze, a bunch of almonds, or a couple of tablespoons of dry oats. Be careful with pre-packaged or industrially accessible smoothies that might be high in fat or normal and fake sugars. Keep your fridge supplied with an assortment of products of the soil, utilize a hard core blender, and make home-made smoothies an everyday custom for your family.

What Are Smoothies

A smoothie is a beverage made from pureed raw
leafy foods/vegetables, ordinarily utilizing
a blender.[A smoothie regularly has a fluid base, for
example, water, organic product juice, plant
milk, and in some cases dairy items
(milk, yogurt, ice-cream, or cottage cheddar).
Smoothies might be made utilizing different fixings
such as crushed

ice, sweeteners (e.g. honey, sugar, stevia,
or syrup), whey powder, nuts, nut margarine,
seeds, tea, chocolate, herbal supplements,
or nutritional supplements.

A smoothie using dairy milk is like a milkshake,
which ordinarily has no or fewer foods grown from
the ground cream or frozen yogurt. As items
ordinarily utilizing crude organic products or
vegetables, smoothies include dietary
fibber (e.g. pulp, skin, and seeds) as are thicker

than fruit juice, regularly with a consistency like a milkshake. Smoothies, especially "green smoothies" that incorporate vegetables, may be marketed to wellbeing cognizant individuals for being more advantageous than milkshakes.

The refreshment of a smoothie relies upon its fixings and their extents. Numerous smoothies incorporate enormous or different servings of products of the soil, which are suggested in a sound eating regimen and proposed to be a meal replacement.

 However, organic product juice containing high sums of sugar can increase caloric intake and promote weight gain. Similarly, fixings such as protein powders, sweeteners, or ice cream are regularly utilized in smoothie recipes, some of which contribute for the most part to season and further caloric intake green smoothie typically comprises of 40–half green vegetables (generally half), usually raw green verdant vegetables, such as spinach, kale, swiss chard, collard greens, celery, parsley, or broccoli, with the rest of the fixings being for the most part or entirely fruit. Wheatgrass and spirulina are additionally utilized as energizing fixings.

Most green verdant vegetables have a bitter flavour when served crude, yet this can be enhanced by picking certain less-harsh vegetables (for example infant spinach) or joining with the certain organic products (e.g. banana softens both the flavour and texture). Some blender manufacturers presently explicitly focus on their items towards making green smoothies and give a booklet of plans to them.

 If the organic product fixings and the green vegetable fixings are both juiced ahead of time, the blended juice doesn't need to be mixed like a smoothie, for example a green juice.

A wide range of smoothies is part
of Indian, Mediterranean, and Middle Eastern
cooking. Fruit sharbat (a famous West and South
Asian beverage) now and again
include yogurt and honey, as well. In India,
the lassi is a smoothie
or milkshake comprising crushed ice, yogurt,
sometimes sugar, and often mango; in
the south, pineapple smoothies made with squashed
ice, sugar, and no yogurt are progressively well
known.

Health food stores on the West Coast of the United States began selling smoothies during the 1930s related to the development of the electric blender.

The genuine term "smoothie" was being utilized in recipes and trademarks by the mid-1980s. Smoothies are an incredible method to devour vegetables in their crude and most nutritious structure, and dissimilar to squeezing, the fibre substance of the fixings in the smoothie is held, bringing about a more beneficial and all the more fulfilling drink.

History Of Smoothies

The History of Smoothies A smoothie is a thick beverage made in a blender. Smoothies for the most part contain products or the like, and may likewise contain different fixings, for example, milk, soy milk, yogurt, dessert, and wholesome enhancements.

 As of late, smoothies have delighted in a lift in prominence because of their notoriety for being sound, however, this beverage has really been around since the mid-twentieth century.

Blending natural products with ice has for quite some time been training in numerous societies. Latin Americans, whose area of the world is renowned for its abundance of tropical natural products, drink a wide range of organic product juice blends.

 These were the motivation for a portion of the main smoothies made in the United States. In India, natural products, for example, mangoes and strawberries are mixed with yogurt and ice to make a beverage called a lassi.

The expression "smoothie" has been around since the mid-twentieth century, yet it wasn't until 1930 that it was utilized to depict a beverage. Early smoothies were just organic products, natural product squeeze, and ice, and they were a dark idea in the United States until the normal food furor of the '60s and '70s.

During these decades, wellbeing food hides away up around the nation, and these stores regularly made and sold mixed natural product drinks.

Blenders - The history of the smoothie is intently attached to the historical backdrop of the blender because without this apparatus, smoothie making would be practically incomprehensible.

The Waring Blender, which was created in the late '30s, was the main blender to be utilized in smoothie making.

More as of late, the presence of the Vita-Mix has upset the universe of smoothies. This blender is sufficiently amazing to granulate fixings like crude vegetables and nuts into a smooth glue, which makes it ideal for making smoothies. In 1973, Steve Kuhnau established the principal Smoothie King in

Louisiana. Kuhnau, who had been exploring different avenues regarding smoothie plans for quite a long time, included fixings, for example, yogurt, protein powder, and nutrients to his smoothies.

Throughout the following three decades, Smoothie King smoothie bars spread the nation over and made the expression "smoothie" a family word.

Simultaneously, smoothies were opening up in more cafés, juice bars, and wellbeing food stores.

Before long, pre-packaged smoothies, made by organizations like Naked Juice and Odwalla, showed up in supermarkets. Today, smoothies of each flavour and assortment are anything but difficult to locate, regardless of where you live.

Also, numerous sites and books offer plans for home-made smoothies.

Assortments - Pretty much anything can be made into a smoothie. Some smoothie producers include vegetables, for example, spinach, carrots, kelp and even hot peppers to make their smoothies extra sound.

You can likewise discover chocolate, vanilla, and espresso smoothies in numerous spots. A portion of these smoothies may appear to be increasingly like milkshakes, yet generally, smoothies contain solid fixings, for example, nutrients and protein powder, and are regularly lower in fat than other velvety beverages

Are Smoothies Healthy

Smoothie has a healthy sparkle about them. They are regularly an essential piece of rinses, and they are universal at health food stores and wellbeing driven cafés.

What is more, the smoothie pattern is yet going solid. Exercise studios serve them up post-class, dietitians lecture their forces and fit celebrities tout their nourishing ability.

However, are smoothies healthy? Some are healthy while some are not. Smoothies made absolutely of entire foods grown from the ground, and whenever wanted, a little soymilk or non-fat dairy, are magnificently sound and nutritious. In any case, in case you are attempting to shed pounds, be cautious.

This is what you should think about the beverage, regardless of whether you are getting one or making your own.

You can put about anything into a smoothie. Be that as it may, most comprise of fluid (like water, non-dairy milk or kefir), natural products, vegetables, seeds, nuts (or nut margarine), supplements like protein powder, maca or matcha, and garnishes, (for example, granola, coconut, and cacao nibs).

The way to making it solid is to find harmony of vegetables, organic product, protein, and fat. The smoothie is an extremely incredible approach to get in those key nourishments.

At the point when you make this kind of smoothie, you have the establishment for a sound breakfast or bite.

Protein can emerge out of unsweetened nut spread, chia, hemp or flax seeds, plain yogurt, or nut milk.

What is more, fat, which helps top you off, is the other key factor in a smoothie. Great wellsprings of fat in smoothies are salt and without sugar nut margarine, chia, flax, sesame, or hemp seeds, flax oil, coconut meat, coconut yogurt, or full-fat natural yogurt,

Also, do grasp assortment. Attempt to stir up the fixings. Dietary assorted variety can be extremely useful to guarantee a balanced supplement consumption.

If you use kale, kefir, and blueberries multi-week, for example, attempt spinach, hemp milk, and pineapple.

Are natural product smoothies healthy?

While natural products have cell reinforcement and mitigating benefits, smoothies regularly become hyper-concentrated wellsprings of organic product sugars. Equalization by including dim verdant

greens like spinach, kale, or Swiss chard (which gives fibre, calcium, nutrients A, C, and K, just as ground-breaking phytochemicals) and protein to hold glucose under tight restraints and control desires and appetite.

Simply be careful with the smoothies you purchase. With locally acquired smoothies, you lose complete command over the quality and amount of the fixings utilized.

Locally acquired assortments may utilize fake sugars, organic product juice, a lot of fat, or improved dairy items, adding to higher measures of sugar, fat, and calories.

Smoothie bowls can likewise contain a lot of sweet granola and improved coconut chips.

Food addictions are genuine addictions with an ever-increasing number of individuals getting snared. Sometimes, these are anything but a significant concern however if these kinds of smoothies are in your customary turn, they could prompt inordinate sugar admission or stomach related trouble.

Are green smoothies sound?

Green smoothies are an incredible method to get necessary vegetables. Just 9% of Americans get the suggested day by day measure of vegetables (2 to 3 cups), regardless of research recommending that plant-based weight control plans diminish the danger of interminable sickness and malignant growth.

Green, verdant vegetables specifically are connected to a lower danger of creating type-2 diabetes, just as more slow age-related intellectual decay. A bunch or two of greens for the most part makes for the best-tasting smoothie.

Are smoothies useful for weight reduction?

Smoothies are regularly touted as an eating regimen food and an approach to detox the body. In any case, with regards to the possibility of a "detox," most specialists concur that smoothies (or some other food, so far as that is concerned) aren't the arrangement — and that the human body has its own assets (to be specific the liver, kidneys, and framework) to purify itself normally.

There's additionally no strong logical proof to propose the possibility of detox for by and large wellbeing or prosperity.

Reasons You Should Drink Smoothie Daily

Still dubious about the medical advantages of smoothies? It is a great opportunity to change that.

Smoothies bode well—for everybody. While a smoothie will never supplant a seared salmon filet with a side of steamed broccoli, it's unquestionably a quick and simple approach to stick protein and vegetables into your eating regimen and harvest the healthful abundance that you might be absent from your different dinners.

Also, on the off chance that you need to lose pounds, drinking smoothies as supper substitutions can be a helpful and delectable approach to altogether slice handled starches and the calories that accompany them.

Studies show that individuals who substitutes breakfast and supper with a high-protein smoothie shed more than 18 pounds in 12 weeks.

Made right, smoothies are brimming with water, fibre, and protein, all which advance "satiety," or feeling full, and can help abstain from indulging and cut calories.

Yet, smoothies brag a tumbler brimming with other medical advantages past weight reduction, contingent upon the fixings you hurl in the blender before the cutting edges begin turning.

Attempt the smoothie plans beneath and see 10 astounding motivations to drink smoothies. Prepare to prepare a scrumptious shake that will do your body great.

1   *Boost Metabolism*

Studies have indicated that including hot fixings like ginger and cayenne pepper to a shake can fire up your calorie-consuming digestion, individuals who devoured about a large portion of a teaspoon of cayenne pepper in their food consumed around 10 additional calories in the hours thereafter, compare with individuals who ate a similar feast yet without the zest.

Analysts call capsaicin, the compound in peppers that makes them hot, a thermogenic synthetic that warms the body, yet diminishes hunger flags in the mind.

Tropical Spice Smoothie

½ cup of coconut water

2 tablespoons new lemon juice

½ ready avocado

1 scoop vanilla whey protein powder

¼ teaspoon cayenne

2" handle of new ginger

1 cup of solidified mango.

Makes 2 servings.

2 *Ease Arthritis Pain*

Throbbing from osteoarthritis-related knee torment? Muscles sore after a quality preparing exercise. Attempt a smoothie made with tart cherry juice, which has been appeared to diminish aggravation and joint agony.

Formula: Almond Cherry Bomb Smoothie

½ cup solidified bing fruits

½ cup tart cherry juice

1 cup Greek yogurt

2 tablespoons almond spread

Makes 2 servings.

3   Reduce Alzheimer's Risk

A few investigations have recommended a potential connection between eating blueberries and improved memory and a decreased danger of Alzheimer's infection.

Researchers accept the anthocyanin cancer prevention agents in blueberries may secure neurons, improve synapse correspondence, and upgrade blood flow to the cerebrum.

This smoothie formula contains different fixings (spinach and turmeric) known to help psychological capacity, settling on it a shrewd decision for boosting mental aptitude.

Formula: The Einstein Smoothie

1 cup solidified blueberries

1 cup of water

½ cup spinach

½ cup Greek yogurt, plain

1 teaspoon matcha powder

½ teaspoon turmeric

¼ cup of coconut milk

ice varying

4. *Revamp Your Gut After Taking Antibiotics*

Anti-infection agents make a great deal of inadvertent blow-back simultaneously they are annihilating the bacterium they are endorsed to slaughter.

They pulverize a lot of our supportive gut microbiota, which thus causes gentle the runs. Yet, now and then the across the board decrease in microbiota by anti-microbials permits a progressively destructive bug–Clostridium difficile—to dominate.

Clostridium-difficile can cause extreme runs and even dangerous irritation of the colon. It is particularly perilous in the old.

There's clinical proof that repopulating the gut with "great bugs" by taking probiotics could help forestall Clostidium-difficle in individuals taking anti-infection agents. Kefir, utilized in the great gut-bug-building smoothie underneath, is probably the best probiotic (yogurt is another) and ideal for smoothie mixes.

Formula: Gut Punch Smoothie

½ cup plain full-fat kefir

1 cup solidified raspberries, peaches, strawberries

½ tablespoon flaxseeds

Makes 1 serving.

5   *Crush Cravings*

Apple juice vinegar and cinnamon have been appeared to settle glucose and save longings for carbs under control.

Formula: Cinnamon and Cider Smoothie

1/3 cup coconut water

1 tablespoon apple juice vinegar

1 teaspoon vanilla concentrate

½ cup plain Greek yogurt

½ teaspoon cinnamon

½ apple, cleaved

four ice

Makes 2 servings.

6. *Lower Blood Pressure*

Eating nourishments wealthy in potassium is a characteristic method to bring down circulatory strain because the mineral tempers the impacts of sodium on the body and furthermore facilitates pressure on vein dividers.

 Among the best high-potassium elements for smoothies are bananas. One investigation found that eating two bananas daily can drop circulatory strain by 10 percent.

However, before you go primate with bananas, check with your primary care physician. Potassium can be hurtful to individuals with kidney issues, and it might collaborate with specific prescriptions.

At that point attempt this circulatory strain bringing down a smoothie, which additionally contains nutrient C, an incredible cancer prevention agent that kills free radicals and loosens up the dividers of your veins.

Formula: Berries and Banana Smoothie

½ cup almond milk

½ cup strawberries, cut

½ medium solidified banana

1 kiwi, stripped and hacked

1 teaspoon ground flaxseeds

Makes 2 servings

7   *Beat Diabetes*

On the off chance that you are stressed over prediabetes, this is a perfect breakfast smoothie to supplant a bowl of sweet grain or improved yogurt.

It poses a flavour like a crusty fruit-filled treat, yet it keeps glucose levels stable with cinnamon, eight grams of fibre, and muscle-building protein.

Likewise, it contains EGCG, catechin from matcha powder that invigorates cells to discharge fat.

Formula: Apple Cobbler Smoothie

1 apple, cored and hacked

1 cup kale, deveined

1 cup unsweetened almond milk

1 teaspoon matcha powder

1 scoop plain plant-based protein powder

cinnamon and nutmeg to taste

Makes 1 serving.

8   *Look Younger*

This smoothie is a dermatologists' most loved because it's stacked with beta-carotene, which the body changes over to nutrient A. This nutrient shields the skin from UV beam harm, conceivably keeping skin graceful and energetic looking. The beta-carotene in this smoothie originates from two fixings, carrots, and apricot.

Honey and cinnamon are included as they have additionally been appeared to help with skin fix.

Formula:

½ cup ground carrot

1 dried apricot half, diced

1 new apricot, hollowed and cleaved

1 teaspoon neighbourhood nectar

1 teaspoon cinnamon

Makes 2 servings.

9   *Stay Awake*

A smoothie made with chilled espresso or cold-blend espresso, banana, and protein powder will not just give you a jolt of energy at 10 a.m., yet it will additionally keep your tummy filled until noon.

Formula:

½ mug espresso cooled or cold blend espresso

½ cup 2% milk

2 Tbsp characteristic nutty spread

1 medium solidified banana

1 scoop whey protein powder

4 ice cubes. Makes 2 servings.

Fruits and tart cherry juice are concentrated wellsprings of melatonin, a famous normal tranquilizer.

Attempt this straightforward mixture as a late-night bite, and you will float off without any problem.

Formula: The Snoozy Smoothie

¾ cup tart cherry juice

1 cup vanilla Greek yogurt

4 ice solid shapes

Makes 2 servings.

Best Fruits for Weight Loss Smoothies

Skirt the sugar and normally improve your mixes with these fundamental, nutrient pressed turbochargers.

With regards to the stars of your smoothie, you most likely have similar main events each time: ice 3d shapes, protein, and a sugar, likely low-sugar, and an organic product.

Yet, imagine a scenario where you could have all that in addition to cancer prevention agents, nutrient C, solid fats, carotenoids, and different supplements that lead to a more extended, more beneficial, more joyful life—without hurling in a Flintstone's nutrient. Blend and match any of these astonishing 8 superfruits to juice yourself dainty.

1 Mango

Nourishment: (1 cup) 103 calories, 24 g sugar, 3 g fibre

This tropical fortune has gotten progressively accessible in American grocery stores, in both new and solidified structures.

Indeed, it's higher in sugar than practically some other natural product in the produce area, however, it additionally brings to the blender 75% of your day's nutrient C and 25 percent of your nutrient A. Consider included sugars totally pointless when making smoothies with mango.

2 *Papaya*

Sustenance: (1 cup) 55 calories, 8 g sugar, 3 g fibre

Is there any organic product preferable for you over papaya? Overwhelmed with nutrient C, packed with vision-fortifying nutrient A, and favoured with one of the greatest fibre-to-sugar proportions conceivable, papaya demonstrates itself to be one of the most balanced nourishments on earth.

Papaya additionally flaunts papain and chymopapain, two intense compounds that have been appeared to battle aggravation, the reason for asthma, joint inflammation, and different genuine conditions.

3 *Blueberries*

Sustenance: (1 cup) 84 calories, 15 g sugar, 4 g fibre .

Blueberries are most popular in wellbeing hovers for anthocyanins, the phytonutrients that give them their blue-red tint, and their thick cancer prevention agent punch.

 That punch converts into genuine mind food, as blueberries have been found in studies to ensure our noggins against both oxidative pressure and the impacts old enough related mental rot showed in Alzheimer's and dementia.

4 *Strawberries*

Nutrition: (1 cup) 49 calories, 7 g sugar, 3 g fibre

Past the beast portion of nutrient C (calorie for calorie, you'll get more C than you'd find in an orange), strawberries additionally end up being a rich wellspring of phenols, including a similar cerebrum boosting, calming anthocyanins found in blueberries.

They likewise make a case for an uncommon and ground-breaking cell reinforcement called ellagitannin, which has been appeared to give a strong guard against an assortment of tumours.

5 *Banana*

Nourishment: (1 medium) 105 calories, 14 g sugar,

3 g fibre

Indeed, there are natural products with more profound dietary portfolios, however, the unassuming banana fills in as a top pick utility player in the smoothie game.

In addition to the fact that it offers a bunch of hard-to-track down supplements (heart-fortifying potassium, gut-accommodating prebiotics), yet it additionally furnishes smoothies with a reasonable, velvety surface and enough regular pleasantness to guarantee no requirement for included sugar.

Keep a couple of exceptionally ready bananas in the cooler. At the point when you're prepared for a smoothie, cut off the strip and mix away.

6 *Avocado*

Nourishment: (1 medium Haas, stripped and pitted) 227 calories, 21 g fat (3 g sat fat), 9 g fibre

The avocado probably will not be a customary smoothie constituent, yet we are persuaded that it ought to be.

The calories come essentially from monounsaturated fat, the great stuff that ensures your heart and assists beat with sponsorship hunger.

Add to that a great fibre burden and you have the makings of a genuinely fulfilling smoothie. In addition, avocados include an extravagance that causes it to feel like you are binge spending, in any event, when you are definitely not.

7 Pineapple

Sustenance: (1 cup) 82 calories, 16 g sugar, 2 g fibre

Feeling low on vitality? A cup of pineapple may very well be the antitoxin. That is on the grounds that pineapple is probably the best wellspring of manganese, a follow mineral that is basic for vitality creation. A cup gives 76 percent of your day by day suggested admission, making pineapple nature's response to Red Bull.

8 Peach

Sustenance: (1 cup) 60 calories, 13 g sugar, 2 g fibre

Peaches pack lutein and zeaxanthin, incredible carotenoids demonstrated to help shield your peepers from macular degeneration.

 In addition, the impact of beta carotene may help fight off coronary illness and malignant growth.

Ingredients You Should Never Add to Smoothie

They make what could have been a healthy shake into a sugar-laden dessert.

Apple juice. Bee pollen. Agave syrup. Trying to order a healthy smoothie is like trying to put together a LEGO set from a bucket of random pieces: All the parts are bright and shiny, but half of them are just junk.

In fact, the selections at most smoothie shops include plenty of "healthy" add-ons that mostly just add on to your waistline. And with more chains opening every day, you will have even more chances to make a mistake. To decode the menu and start melting your belly for real, take a look at these six worst ingredients to add to your smoothie.

1 Fat-Free Flavoured Yogurt

High in protein with a delicious creamy texture,

yogurt is the ideal backbone for a smoothie—unless it is flavoured or fat-free. Yogurts with fruit on the bottom of mix-ins like honey can contain up to 29 grams of sugar (that is the amount in even a "healthy" brand like Fage Honey Greek Yogurt). Stick to full-fat, plain yogurt.

The more high-fat dairy products people ate, the lower their risk of diabetes; those who ate a lot of low-fat dairy products had the highest incidence.

 The researchers speculated that while calcium, protein, vitamin D, and other nutrients in dairy are indeed good for us, we need the fat that goes along with them in order to get their protective effects. Skipping the fat may cost you lean muscle: "People with low vitamin D levels have been shown to have decreased strength and greater muscle wasting.

2 Fruit Juice

You glance at the blender, worried there's not enough liquid. Don't be tempted to add some leftover or that can of frozen apple concentrate lurking in the freezer: Fruit juices lack the satiating fibre of fresh fruit, and even half a cup of orange juice adds 13 grams of carbs. It is even worse at the smoothie chains.

3 Ice Cream or Sherbet

Smoothies that include ice cream, frozen yogurt or sherbet are not fitness drinks. They are desserts. A small (20 ounce) Berry Punch sounds like something healthy. But because it contains raspberry sherbet, it packs 84 grams of sugar.

A large scoop of unflavoured Greek yogurt and a handful of frozen fruit will give you the same flavour and consistency—without several nights' worth of dessert.

4 Too Much of a Good Thing

Avocado and nut butter are some of your best allies in the pursuit of a flat stomach, but too much of their good fats can backfire. Be mindful of the portions suggested by recipes. Nutritionists consider one-fifth of an avocado to be one serving. Likewise, one serving of nut butter is just two tablespoons and more than enough for a savoury smoothie.

Use almond butter—but to repeat, just two tablespoons. Ounce for ounce, almonds are one of the most nutritious nuts. They're a great source of riboflavin, magnesium, and manganese which is great for the prevention of osteoporosis as well as a healthy metabolism, and also provides an impressive amount of vitamin E per serving. You'll also get flavonoids, compounds that are extremely useful in fighting heart disease and cancer.

5 Added Sweeteners

You would not dare add straight granulated sugar to your smoothies (right?), but other healthy-sounding additives don't act so sweet, either. A tablespoon of all-natural honey will add 17 grams of sugar to your drink, while a similar serving of virtuous-sounding agave nectar will add an unnecessary five grams.

And while a serving of coconut oil is an excellent add-in — its good saturated fats are burned as energy, not stored as fat — other variations on that tropical theme are trouble.

Coconut nectar, increasingly common at smoothie bars, will add 13 grams of sugar and carbs per tablespoon, and sweetened coconut flakes have an eye-popping 24 grams of fat and 36 grams of sugars per cup.

For sweetness, rely on whole fruit and sugar-free almond milk—and for an eye-opening look at what artificial sweetener and corn syrup can do to you.

6 Canned Fruit

Canned fruit might seem like an easy shortcut, but it is just a quick route to belly fat. It is packed with syrup — upwards of 20 grams of sugars a can! — and nasty additives such as artificial flavourings.

Even unsweetened fruit in its own juice is a nutritional miss: Peeled fruit is missing crucial fibre, and vitamin content can degrade in the canning process.

If having fresh fruit around the house for your smoothies is impractical, go for frozen—they add a frosty texture and freezing preserves more nutrients than canning does because the frozen ones are picked then immediately (or soon after) frozen.
  Just read the labels on frozen packages to make sure there are no added sodium, sugar, or chemicals.

Things To Add To Your Smoothies For Quicker Weight Loss

There is an explanation smoothie is cherished by health monstrosities around the globe. They are anything but difficult to make and are a snappy breakfast fix for individuals who are generally in a hurry toward the beginning of the day. And you can add nearly anything to them.

 They are the ideal energize drinks for your post-exercise suppers and smoothie plans are entirely manageable to a wide range of new and solid fixings, from berries to new organic products, vegetables, protein, and oat powders, just as sound nuts and seeds.

Smoothies are favoured beverages for individuals hoping to shed pounds on account of the effortlessly altered nature of the beverage.

Aside from adding nutritious superfoods to your morning meal smoothie, you can likewise include the accompanying fat-consuming nourishments to accomplish brisk weight reduction:

1. Green Tea Powder

Green tea is notable for its weight reduction
advancing forces. Adding green tea powder to your
smoothie can trigger the arrival of fat from your
cells, because of the catechins present in it.
 Green tea doesn't have any overwhelming flavour,
so you needn't stress over it ruining the taste either.

2. Blueberries and Strawberries

These minuscule powerhouses ought to never be
thought little of. Blueberries have demonstrated
their strength as incredible fat terminators in various
examinations.

 They are loaded with cell reinforcements and are fit
for initiating qualities that consume fat.
Strawberries are stars in their own correct with
regards to weight reduction. They have polyphenols
that can stop the arrangement of fat in the body.

3. Spinach

A verdant green in your smoothie does not sound
appealing, however, recall, the objective here is to

trigger fat consumption. Spinach is perhaps the best thing to add to your smoothie as a result of its

ability to satisfy you for longer by providing fibre to your body.

4. Coconut Oil

Coconut oil is an assigned superfood whose widespread intrigue continues rising. Studies have discovered that eating two teaspoons of coconut oil can bring about loss of midsection fat. Besides, coconut oil does not have a very remarkable taste or enhance and henceforth, can be placed in any beverage you like.

5. Cinnamon

Cinnamon is the supported flavour of individuals needing to get in shape quickly, all around the globe. It eases swelling and solutions for water maintenance. Aside from this, it additionally upgrades the kind of beverage.

6. Chia Seeds

Developed basically for the oil, chia seeds have immovably made their place in the classification of solid nourishments, with individuals utilizing them around the globe. Chia seeds help in expanding the satiety factor of your beverage, forestalling cravings for food and your need to nibble often.

7. Flaxseeds

Flaxseeds, otherwise called alsi ka beej in Hindi is one of the most astonishing weight reduction fixings out there. Flaxseeds are an extraordinary wellspring of solvent adhesive (gum like) fibre that can bring down terrible cholesterol in the blood. They likewise go about as craving suppressants.

8. Beetroots

Beetroots are perfect wellbeing nourishments because of their rich supplement profile, yet they have an incredible task to carry out in weight reduction as well. They are wealthy in cancer prevention agents and low in calories and sugar. They have additionally been known to support muscle capacity to assist you with working out better.

9. Oats Powder

Powdered oats are constantly added to breakfast smoothies to make them more filling. Oats are wealthy in fibre and subsequently can assist you with saving full for more, forestalling desires or pigging out.

10. Ginger/Ginger Powder

The magnificent Asian root ginger or adrak is additionally an Ayurvedic superfood with various medical advantages. It can help your digestion and furthermore balance glucose levels, shielding you from needing to overeat.

Other than these, there are a ton of other sound and nutritious natural products, vegetables, flavours, and herbs you can add to your smoothies, contingent upon the amount you are willing to mess with taste and flavours.

60 Super Healthy Smoothies For Weight Loss

Smoothies can absolutely be a part of your strategy for wellbeing, lasting weight loss—if that is what you are after—but only when done right. (Otherwise, consider them slurpable desserts with a health halo around them.) Nutritionists agree that incorporating a nutrient-dense smoothie into your daily diet can help avoid pound creepage by keeping hunger levels in check and even promote weight loss thanks to their filling fibre and muscle-building protein.

Before we get into those, let us chat about weight loss for a minute. A perfect smoothie will not magically make you lose weight. In fact, no one thing is going to do that—at least not in a healthy or sustainable way. If you want to lose weight (and not everyone does), you must also address a range of other factors that play important roles: sleep, stress, hormones, and other medical issues, to name a few biggies.

Only by looking at weight loss from a holistic point of view can you home in on a healthy goal, effect meaningful change, and see sustainable results. For some people, weight loss in and of itself might not be a healthy goal. If you have a history of disordered eating, you should consult a doctor before making any changes to your diet.

Now, whether you're looking for help on your road to weight loss or just want some delectable smoothie inspiration, read on, and dust off that blender as you set to embrace this 60 amazing healthy weight loss smoothies.

1

Pumpkin Powerhouse

What gives pumpkins their gorgeous orange colour is the antioxidant beta-carotene. This nutrient is helpful in slowing down aging in the body. Did we mention pumpkin is a rich source of vitamin C? With only 49 calories, a cup of cooked pumpkin boasts 3 grams of fibre—great for filling you up without weighing you down.

Ingredients:

1 cup pumpkin puree (canned or fresh)
1 cup unsweetened vanilla almond milk
1/2 frozen banana (adds creaminess and sweetness without added sugar)

a handful of ice cubes
dash of pumpkin pie spice (swap for cinnamon if
you don't have this)
Blend all ingredients together and enjoy.

2

Green Sunrise Smoothie
The Green Sunrise Smoothie has everything you
need to start your day right, you'll get a healthy
dose of omega-3 fatty acids and essential vitamins
and minerals to keep you healthy and strong while
losing weight."

Ingredients:
1 scoop protein powder (Miller uses Medifast's
Pineapple Mango Smoothie packet)
1 cup fresh spinach
1½ oz sliced avocado
1 cup unsweetened almond or cashew milk
1 tbsp ground flaxseed
Blend all ingredients together and enjoy.

3

Chia-Berry Belly Blaster
 This creamy, decadent smoothie is also a nutrient
powerhouse with the addition of chia seeds and
berries. This super simple smoothie is packed full

of protein and fibre to crush cravings and keep you feeling satisfied for hours. The omega-3 fatty acids in the chia seeds help reduce stress hormones and decrease inflammation, and the berries are packed full of antioxidants.

Ingredients:
1 cup plain Greek yogurt, unsweetened
1 cup frozen berries (blueberries, strawberries, or açai berries make great options)
1 tbsp vanilla extract
1 tbsp ground chia seeds
1/2 cup ice
Blend all ingredients together and enjoy.

4

Spicy Tropical Greens Delight
Capsaicin, the active ingredient found in peppers, acts as a mild metabolism stimulant. As a bonus, pineapple has a diuretic effect which helps the body get rid of retained water. Did we mention how good all the phytochemicals, vitamins, and minerals found in those greens are? Yeah.

Ingredients:
1 cup frozen mango chunks
1 cup frozen pineapple chunks
1 1/2 unsweetened coconut water
1 cup leafy greens (baby spinach, kale, collard

greens, etc.)
1/4 cup lime juice
1/4 tsp cayenne pepper (optional)
Blend all ingredients together and enjoy. (Note:
This recipe yields about two servings.)

5

Vanilla-Berry Blast
At just 250 calories, this refreshing and delicious
smoothie is packed with 18 grams of protein and 5
grams of fibre to keep you satisfied and to keep
energy and blood sugar level on an even keel
without crashes.

 The rich and creamy sweetness of this smoothie is
especially great to satisfy a sweet tooth if you are
trying to avoid consuming extra calories from
unhealthier options. Plus, the berries contain the
phytochemical C3G that may increase the
production of both adiponectin (which enhances fat
metabolism) and leptin (which suppresses appetite).

Ingredients:
1 quart plain non-fat Greek yogurt
8 ounces unsweetened frozen strawberries or
blueberries
2 cups unsweetened vanilla almond milk
1 banana, frozen
1 tsp cinnamon
Add half of each of the yogurt, berries, and milk
into a blender and blend until smooth. Add the
remainder of the ingredients and blend until smooth.

(Note: This recipe yields about three servings so either refrigerate for later or pour into three glasses and share!)

6

Spirulina Smoothie
 The low-calorie superfood is brimming with nutrients and is an easy slip-in for your next shake or smoothie bowl. A 500 mg serving contains just 2 calories, allowing you to pack your body with nutrients while saving on calories.

The protein in spirulina is also easily digested and absorbed, making it easier to build lean muscle, which helps the body burn more calories and fat throughout the day.

Ingredients:
1 banana
1/2 cup coconut water
1/2 cup almond milk
1 scoop vegan vanilla protein powder (optional)
1 tsp spirulina
Blend all ingredients together and enjoy.

7

Tummy Busting Berry Smoothie

Here, velvety banana merges along with digestion boosting berries (blueberries and raspberries contain the flavonoid anthocyanin, which is related to lower glucose levels, fewer longings, and expanded digestion) in a basic shake that is as filling as it is tasty.

The nut spread gives sound fats and protein to keep you fulfilled for a couple of hours and keep blood sugars consistent, this forestalls thoughtless eating on high-sugar, fatty nourishments that add to weight gain. On account of banana's high potassium content, this shake helps squash swelling.

Ingredients:

1 cup almond milk

1 cup solidified berries (strawberries, raspberries, blackberries, and so forth.)

1 banana

1 tbsp almond or nutty spread

bunch of ice

Mix all fixings together and appreciate it.

Green Smoothie

Go green or return home! On the off chance that you are searching for a veggie lover smoothie formula or a solid breakfast smoothie, this green smoothie is pressed with vegetables, sound fats, and is so velvety and scrumptious you'll never take a gander at another green smoothie formula again!

Ingredients:

1 medium solidified avocado

1 cup packed spinach

1 cup sliced solidified banana

1 tablespoon ground flax

1/4 cup frozen cauliflower florets

3 pitted Medjool dates

1.25 cups unsweetened almond milk (or more, to taste mix all elements for your green smoothie until smooth.

9

 Classic Strawberry Smoothie

In under 5 minutes you can have the most heavenly strawberry smoothie formula all set. It's made with 4 basic fixings and the children will adore it.

INGREDIENTS
1.5 cups entire solidified strawberries

1/2 medium banana

1/2 cup plain non-fat Greek yogurt

1 cup 100% squeezed orange

 spot all fixings into a blender and blend on high speed until smooth. The alternative to include somewhat progressively squeezed orange relying upon how thick/dainty you like your smoothies. Serve immediately.

10

Peanut Butter Banana Smoothie

Peanut spread and banana is a fan most loved with regards to enhancing combos. That is the reason this nutty spread banana smoothie formula is a show-halting smoothie formula you must make! We kept this nutty spread and banana smoothie straightforward with only 6 complete fixings!

Ingredients

2 cups solidified cut bananas

1/2 cup non-fat Greek yogurt

1/2 tablespoon ground flax seeds

1 cup unsweetened almond milk

1 teaspoon vanilla extract

2 tablespoons all-normal nutty spread

spot all fixings into a high-speed blender. Mix on high until smooth. Include more almond milk varying. Serve right away.

11

STRAWBERRY BANANA SPINACH SMOOTHIE

Whip up this scrumptious strawberry banana spinach smoothie formula in the blink of an eye with our mystery dinner prep smoothies' stunt! We are telling you the best way to make this stunning and nutritious spinach smoothie promptly or how to make ahead for some other time!

INGREDIENTS

2 cups solidified cut bananas

2 cups solidified entire strawberries

4 cups new spinach

4 teaspoons chia seeds

2 tablespoons vanilla protein powder (any kind)

1/2 cup unsweetened almond milk

Instruction for the bag

First, line a preparing sheet with material paper. At that point, equitably spread out 2 cups of cut bananas, 2 cups of entire strawberries.

A spot in the cooler for around 2 hours or until totally solidified. Next, take 4 quart-size cooler packs and compose the date and Strawberry Banana.

Green Smoothie on the front. Include 1 cup of the solidified natural product, a bunch of spinach, and a teaspoon of chia seeds to each sack. Prior to fixing, ensure you crush however much ventilate as could be expected to forestall cooler consume. Seal and spot in the cooler for later use

12

Triple Berry Protein Smoothie

This Triple Berry Protein Smoothie is pressed with clean fixings and an astounding 12 grams of protein for every serving. Made with blended berries, banana, protein powder, almond milk, and chia seeds, this protein smoothie will begin your day away from work right!

INGREDIENTS

1.5 cups solidified triple berry blend

1 medium solidified banana

1/2 tablespoon chia seeds

1/4 cup vanilla protein powder

1.25 cups unsweetened almond mil

Spot all fixings in a high-speed blender and blend until smooth.

NOTES

Option to include more almond milk by the ¼ cup contingent upon how thick or meagre you like your smoothies.

13

Banana Protein shake

This Healthy Banana Protein Shake is stuffed with a short rundown of genuine fixings and mixed together to flawlessness! Bragging 16 g protein for every serving and very tasty, this protein shake formula will fuel your body post-exercise or as a sweet treat.

INGREDIENTS

¾ cup non-fat Greek yogurt, solidified into 3D shapes

2 cups solidified cut bananas

1 teaspoon vanilla concentrate

¼ cup vanilla protein

2 cups milk, any

NOTES

Contingent upon how thick you like your shakes, the alternative to include more milk by the tablespoon until the wanted thickness is reached.

Nourishment does exclude showered nutty spread or whipped coconut cream toppings

INSTRUCTIONS

In the first place, freeze ¾ cup non-fat Greek Yogurt in an ice 3 shape plate.

When the Greek yogurt has completely solidified, place all elements for sound banana shake into a rapid blender.

Mix until smooth and present with your preferred fixings.

14

STRAWBERRY BANANA SMOOTHIE WITH PEANUT BUTTER

Need to take your exemplary strawberry banana smoothie formula up an indent? Include a couple of tablespoons of nutty spread for an epic wind on a morning meal smoothie

Ingredients

1 cup of solidified strawberries

1 cup solidified cut banana

1/4 cup non-fat plain Greek yogurt

2 tablespoons all-normal velvety nutty spread

1 tablespoon ground flax seeds

1 teaspoon vanilla concentrate

1 cup unsweetened almond milk

Spot all fixings in a fast blender and blend until smooth.

Present with a sprinkle of nutty spread and new organic product.

15

PUMPKIN SMOOTHIE WITH CASHEW BUTTER

Go through your extra canned pumpkin and make this Pumpkin Berry Cashew Butter Smoothie! It joins delightful fall flavours making a yummy superfood-filled breakfast or nibble fixings

Ingredients

2 tablespoons pumpkin puree

1 tablespoon cashew spread

1 cup solidified blueberries

1/2 solidified banana

1/2 tablespoon flaxseed dinner

1/2 teaspoon pumpkin pie flavor

1 cup almond milk, unsweetened

Directions

Spot all fixings in a rapid blender and mix on high until smooth.

Scratch the sides of the blender and include extra almond milk (1 teaspoon at once) if the smoothie is excessively thick. Mix until smooth.

Present with natively constructed granola or natural product garnishes and appreciate it!

CHOCOLATE PROTEIN SHAKE

This chocolate protein shake is chocolatey, pressed with protein, and the ideal post-exercise nibble or simple breakfast formula!

Ingredients

1 cup solidified blueberries

1 medium solidified banana

1/4 cup chocolate protein powder (any sort!)

1 tablespoon cocoa powder

1/4 cup non-fat Greek yogurt

2 tablespoons cashew spread

1/2 tablespoon ground flaxseed

1 cup unsweetened plain almond milk

Directions

Spot all fixings into a rapid blender.

Mix on high for around 1 moment, halting to scratch the sides. You may need to add more milk to thin varying.

Serve right away!

17

The best Pumpkin Smoothie

A tasty pumpkin smoothie made with your morning espresso so you don't need to pick between the two

Fixings

2 medium solidified bananas

1/2 cup unsweetened pumpkin puree

3/4 mug espresso, cold

3/4 cup milk, any sort

1/2 teaspoon pumpkin pie flavour

1 teaspoon maple syrup

Directions

Spot all fixings into a rapid blender.

Mix on high for around 1 moment, halting to scratch the sides if necessary.

Serve quickly with your preferred whipped beating.

18

STRAWBERRY PROTEIN SHAKE

What is superior to cheesecake for breakfast? NOTHING! You are going to cherish this Strawberry Protein Shake since it tastes precisely like strawberry cheesecake. This protein powder smoothie formula is made with only a couple of straightforward fixings: solidified strawberries, bananas, vanilla protein powder, Greek yogurt, and almond milk

Fixings

1.5 cups entire solidified strawberries

1/2 cup solidified cut banana

1/4 cup vanilla protein powder (any thoughtful will work)

1/3 cup non fat Greek yogurt

1 cup unsweetened almond milk

Guidelines

Spot all fixings into a fast blender and mix until smooth. Include more almond milk varying relying upon inclination.

19

BLUEBERRY BANANA SMOOTHIE

This blueberry banana smoothie is the smoothie everything being equal! It is made with solidified natural product, almond milk, flax supper, and a smidgen of vanilla. This blueberry banana smoothie is thick and ideal for a sound breakfast or a delicious snack

INGREDIENTS

1 cup solidified blueberries

1 cup solidified cut bananas

1 tablespoon flax feast

1 cup unsweetened almond milk

1 teaspoon vanilla concentrate

Guidelines

Spot all fixings into a fast blender and mix until smooth.

20 .

THE BEST BREAKFAST SMOOTHIE

Start your day away from work directly with this protein-pressed solid breakfast smoothie. Loaded up with organic product, oats, protein powder, almond milk and a little hit of nutty spread, this morning meal smoothie of all morning meal smoothies will keep you feeling fulfilled till lunch.

INGREDIENTS

1 medium solidified banana

1 cup of solidified strawberries

2 tablespoons moved cereal

¼ cup vanilla protein powder

1 tablespoon all-regular smooth nutty spread

1 cup plain unsweetened almond milk

INSTRUCTIONS : Place everything into a fast blender. Mix on high, halting to scratch the sides varying, until smooth.

Serve right away!

21 .

PEANUT BUTTER GREEN SMOOTH

We present to you, a green smoothie that does not taste green! This nutty spread green smoothie is a fan top pick. It is pressed with protein, greens, and nutty spread goodness

Fixings

2 cups cut solidified bananas

3 tablespoon all-characteristic nutty spread

2 tablespoons salted peanuts

1.5 cups unsweetened almond milk 1 cup spinach, stuffed

Directions

Spot all elements for your smoothie into a rapid blender. Mix on high for 1-2 minutes or until smooth. Alternative to add more almond milk to thin things out varying.

Top with your preferred fixings, for example, nutty spread and simmered peanuts.

22.

BANANA MATCHA SMOOTHIE

Start your three day weekend with this Banana Matcha Smoothie for a supplement stuffed sound breakfast. It is the ideal blend of sweet bananas with gritty matcha just as delectable greens that are wealthy in iron. Trust us, you will be alert and fulfilled throughout the morning!

Fixings

1 cup banana cuts, solidified

1 teaspoon matcha

1 cup new spinach, pressed

2 teaspoons flax seed

1 teaspoon vanilla concentrate

3/4 cup unsweetened almond milk (or more if necessary)

Directions

Spot all fixings in a blender and mix until smooth .

23

DARK CHOCOLATE DATE PROTEIN SMOOTHIE

Longing for a chocolate shake? Make this Dark Chocolate Date Protein Smoothie rather for a similar extraordinary flavour, yet quite a lot more nourishment! With 10g of protein and 9g of fibre, this protein smoothie is the ideal post-exercise titbit or breakfast in a hurry

Fixings

2 solidified bananas, medium

3 medjool dates, pitted

1 cup kale, deboned and hacked

3 tablespoons dull cocoa powder

1/2 teaspoon vanilla concentrate

1 cup nut milk of your decision

Directions

Spot all fixings into a rapid blender and blend until smooth.

24

RICH STRAWBERRY CHIA SEED SMOOTHIE

Start the vacation day directly with this rich strawberry chia seed smoothie! This smoothie is pressed with cancer prevention agents, fibre, and extraordinary flavour! You will not be disillusioned when you include the chia seeds for some additional surface and fun. Mix up this rich strawberry chia seed smoothie today

Fixings

1 cup of solidified strawberries

1 medium banana

1/2 cup plain non-fat Greek yogurt

1 cup almond milk, unsweetened

1/2 teaspoon vanilla concentrate

1 tablespoon chia seeds

Directions

Spot all fixings in a blender and mix until smooth! Let sit for a couple of moments so that the chia seeds can do their enchantment (grow and get vile). Enjoy it!

25

BANANA SMOOTHIE

Let me acquaint you with the creamiest and most scrumptious banana smoothie. This sound banana smoothie is basic and pressed with protein, fibre, and potassium! Mix it up this week for a solid banana smoothie breakfast!

Fixings

2 cups solidified cut bananas

1/2 cup non-fat plain Greek yogurt

1/2 tablespoon ground flax seeds

1 cup unsweetened plain almond milk

1 teaspoon vanilla concentrate

Directions

Spot all fixings in a rapid blender and mix on high speed until smooth. Alternative to include more almond milk varying

26

POMEGRANATE GREEN SMOOTHIE

Get extravagant with your smoothie and make this flavourful pomegranate green smoothie bowl bested with pomegranate arils, pistachios, hemp seeds, and dim chocolate!

Fixings

1/2 cup solidified strawberries

1 solidified banana, medium

1 cup new kale, pressed

1/2 cup Greek yogurt

1/2 cup pomegranate juice

1/2 cup water

1 scoop vanilla protein powder (any sort!)

garnishes: hemp seeds, pomegranate arils, pistachio nuts, and dim chocolate

Guidelines

Spot all fixings in a fast food processor and blend until smooth. You may need to include more pomegranate juice relying upon how thick you like your smoothies.

27

Crusty fruit-filled treat SMOOTHIE BOWL

Love crusty fruit-filled treat? Presently you can have it for breakfast and not feel an ounce of blame! This crusty fruit-filled treat smoothie bowl is made with genuine food and great crusty fruit-filled treat flavour!

Fixings

1 solidified banana, little

1/2 cup non-fat vanilla Greek yogurt*

2/3 cup fruit purée, unsweetened

1/4 cup moved oats

1 teaspoon cinnamon

1 teaspoon vanilla concentrate

1/2 cup almond milk, unsweetened

discretionary: a bunch of new spinach or kale

Guidelines

Spot all fixings in a fast blender. Mix until smooth.

Present with heaps of fixings on top!

28

BLUEBERRY SPINACH SMOOTHIE

Do you need an increase in nutrients or minerals? This blueberry spinach smoothie is pressed with nutrient c to help support your safe framework and keep your body feeling great!

Fixings

1 huge banana

1 cup non fat Greek yogurt

1 cup new blueberries

2 cups stuffed spinach

1 cup 100% squeezed orange

1 teaspoon new ginger, stripped and ground

2–3 cups of ice

Directions

Spot all fixings in a rapid blender and blend until smooth

29

NUTTY SPREAD AND JELLY PROTEIN SMOOTHIE

This nutty spread and jam protein smoothie is a scrumptious and sound turn on your preferred youth great. Besides, it is the ideal post-exercise nibble stuffed with protein and unbelievably delicious.

.INGREDIENTS

1 cup blended solidified berries

1–2 tablespoons all-regular nutty spread

1/4 cup vanilla protein powder

2 tablespoons moved oats

1 cup milk, any sort

Directions

Spot all fixings in a blender and blend until smooth

30

APPLE SMOOTHIE

This apple smoothie formula is a superb solid breakfast thought or titbits. It is made with solidified fruit purée, almond milk, ground flaxseed, and your preferred nut spread

Fixings

2 4-oz. fruit purée cups, frozen

1 cup unsweetened almond milk (or any sort of milk)

2 tablespoons moved oats

2 tablespoons nut margarine (any sort)

1 teaspoon ground flax seed

1 teaspoon maple syrup

1/4 teaspoon ground cinnamon

Guidelines

To start with, freeze 2 4-oz. fruit purée cups for at any rate 2 hours or overnight.

When solidified, run the fruit purée cups under high temp water for a couple of moments to expel from the plastic. At that point place into a rapid blender.

Include the remainder of the fixings and spread.

Mix on high for around a moment or until smooth.

31

STRAWBERRY PINEAPPLE SMOOTHIE

Get a spoon and make this thick and tasty Strawberry Pineapple Smoothie with only a couple of sound fixings.

Fixings

1.5 cups solidified pineapple pieces

1.5 cups solidified strawberries

1/2 cup vanilla Greek yogurt

1 teaspoon vanilla concentrate

1.5 cups almond milk, unsweetened (or more to taste)

Directions

Spot all elements for your strawberry pineapple smoothie into a rapid blender.

Mix on high until smooth. Contingent upon how solidified your natural product is, you may need to include more almond milk.

Present with extra new pineapple pieces on the base.

32

ORANGE CREAMSICLE SMOOTHIE

Searching for the orange smoothie you had always wanted? Attempt our enchanted nutrient C-stuffed Orange Creamsicle Smoothie. You just need 3 fixings + a couple nummy include ins!

Fixings

1 cup solidified banana cuts

1 teaspoon vanilla concentrate

1 cup 100% squeezed orange

discretionary: 1/2 cup ice

discretionary: 1 scoop vanilla protein powder, coconut whipped cream, orange pizzazz

Guidelines

Spot solidified bananas, vanilla concentrate, and squeezed orange into a rapid blender and mix until smooth.

Choice now to include a bunch of ice (contingent upon thickness inclination) and additionally other include ins, for example, vanilla protein powder and new orange get-up-and-go.

Mix once again and afterward serve right away.

33

CHOCOLATE PEANUT BUTTER SMOOTHIE

This nutty spread cup smoothie is stuffed with protein and even has a full serving of greens in it. The best part is, it's solid and tastes precisely like a nutty spread cup!

Fixings

2 cups cut solidified bananas

3 tablespoons all-characteristic rich nutty spread

1/4 cup cocoa powder

1 tablespoon ground flaxseed

1 cup pressed spinach

1 cup almond milk

Guidelines

Expel solidified bananas from the cooler and spot them into a rapid blender.

Next, include the remainder of the fixings to the blender and mix until smooth.

On the off chance that the smoothie is excessively thick, gradually include a tablespoon of almond milk at once until smoothie arrives at wanted consistency.

34

MANGO SMOOTHIE RECIPE

This 4-fixing solid smoothie is prepared to appreciate in a short time or less and makes the ideal breakfast or titbit.

Fixing

2 cups solidified mango cuts

1 15-oz. can light coconut milk

1/2 tablespoon flaxseed dinner

1 huge solidified banana

Directions

Spot the entirety of the fixings into a fast blender.

Mix on high until smooth.

Eat right away.

35

 KALE SMOOTHIE

Get your everyday greens here! This is the most flavourful kale smoothie you will ever make! It is pressed with supplement thick kale, solidified bananas, and the ideal flavour punch of squeezed orange and new ginger. Prepare this green smoothie in a short time and you're making excellent progress so far with a sound breakfast or nibble in a hurry.

Fixings

2 cups solidified bananas

2 cups stuffed slashed kale

1 tablespoon flax dinner

2 Medjool dates pitted

discretionary: 1/2 teaspoon new ground ginger

1.5 cups squeezed orange

Directions

Spot all fixings in a fast blender and mix on high until smooth. Alternative to include progressively squeezed orange varying.

36

 Carrot Cake Smoothie

This straightforward and simple Carrot Cake Smoothie is the ideal breakfast or nibble and an extraordinary, sound, approach to fulfil your sweet tooth!

Fixings

8 pecans

1 huge carrot, generally slashed (or ground in the event that you don't have a fast blender)

An extra finely ground carrot for blending in, discretionary

1 teaspoon of cinnamon

A sprinkle of nutmeg, newly ground is EXTRA flavourful

2 pitted dates

½–1 cup of fluid, I ordinarily use non-dairy milk and afterward include water on the off chance that I need it more liquidly

1 teaspoon of vanilla

½ of a solidified banana

Directions

In a rapid blender, mix all fixings (less the extra carrot) together until velvety and smooth.

Whenever wanted, blend in extra finely ground carrot (energetically suggest!). Top with a couple of slashed pecans.

37

Blueberry Date Shake

Blueberry Date Shake. A rich and velvety solid veggie lover "milkshake" made without frozen yogurt. The formula utilizes dates, almond milk, and any of your preferred organic product.

Fixings

2 medium bananas — cut into pieces and solidified (around 8 ounces or 1/2 cups cut)

1 cup solidified blueberries — around 4 ounces

3 pitted Medjool dates — in addition to extra taste

1 tablespoon almond spread — in addition to extra taste

1/2 teaspoon unadulterated vanilla concentrate

1 cup Almond Breeze almond milk Unsweetened Vanilla

2-3 ice 3D shapes — discretionary

Directions

Spot the banana, blueberries, dates, almond spread, vanilla concentrate, and almond milk in a powerful blender (on the off chance that you don't have a powerful blender.

38

Beet Smoothie

Blueberry Beet Smoothie. Sweet, smooth, and stuffed with fibre, protein, and cancer prevention agents! This solid breakfast smoothie is ideal for weight reduction or for kids. Flavourful, fruity, and the beets are not excessively solid.

Fixings

1/2 cup unsweetened almond milk or milk of decision

1 cup blended solidified blueberries or blended berries

1 little beet — stripped and diced (around 8 ounces)

1/4 cup solidified pineapple

1/4 cup plain non-fat Greek yogurt — use non-dairy yogurt to make vegetarian

Discretionary sugar: 1-2 teaspoons nectar — in addition to extra to taste (use agave to make veggie lover)

Discretionary blend ins: chia seeds — hempseed, or potentially ground flaxseed (I like mine with a sprinkle of chia or hempseed) I additionally prefer to add 2 tablespoons oats to make the smoothie considerably all the more filling.

Directions

Spot the almond milk, blueberries, beet, pineapple, and Greek yogurt in a rapid blender, for example, a Vitamix (on the off chance that you don't have a fast blender, I'd recommend microwaving, simmering, or daintily steaming the beets before utilizing with the goal that they are milder and puree all the more easily).

Mix until smooth. Taste and on the off chance that you want a better smoothie, include somewhat nectar or date and mix once more.

Appreciate promptly or refrigerate for up to 1 day. blending the milk and half of the solidified natural product first, at that point easing back including the remainder of the leafy foods fixings). Mix until smooth.

If you might want the shake somewhat thicker, include a couple of ice shapes and mix once more. Taste and include extra almond spread on the off chance that you would like the shake a little more extravagant or another date on the off chance that you'd like it better. Pour and enjoy it!

39

Berry Turmeric Smoothie

Berry Turmeric Smoothie with blueberry, spinach, ginger, and nectar. An ideal solid breakfast smoothie to launch your mornings! This simple smoothie is extraordinary for kids since you cannot taste or see the green. Other medical advantages incorporate going about as a characteristic insusceptible supporter, cold cure, and against aggravation drink.

Fixings

3/4 cup unsweetened vanilla almond milk — or milk of decision

2 cups child spinach — around 2 huge bunches

1/2 cup non fat plain Greek yogurt — or without dairy yogurt of decision

3 tablespoons antiquated moved oats

1/2 cups solidified blended berries — I utilized a mix of blackberries, blueberries, and raspberries

1/2 teaspoon Ground Turmeric

1/4 teaspoon Ground Ginger

2-3 teaspoons nectar — or trade agave or maple syrup to make veggie lover, in addition to extra to taste

Guidelines

Spot the fixings in a powerful blender in the request recorded: almond milk, spinach, yogurt, oats, berries, turmeric, ginger, and 2 teaspoons nectar. Mix until smooth. Taste and change pleasantness as wanted. If you don't have a powerful blender, I suggest mixing the almond milk, spinach, and yogurt first, and afterward including different fixings. Enjoy right away

40

Coconut Chocolate Mint Chip Smoothie

This chocolate mint chip smoothie is velvety, thick, and rich gratitude to the coconut and solidified riced cauliflower. It is low in sugar and stacked with protein and sound fats so you will feel fulfilled and your glucose will remain adjusted.

Fixings

1 cup unsweetened almond, cashew or coconut milk

1/2 coconut water (or more milk)

1–2 Tablespoons coconut margarine

1/2–1 cup solidified cauliflower rice

1 scoop chocolate protein powder

1 Tablespoon chia seeds

1/2 Tablespoon cacao or cocoa powder

4–5 new mint leaves or 1–2 drops of peppermint separate

1–2 teaspoons cacao nibs

granola, for garnish (discretionary)

Guidelines

Mix all fixings aside from cacao nibs and granola in a powerful blender

Mix until smooth. Include cacao nibs and mix two or three seconds more. Fill a glass, sprinkle with granola and cacao nibs and enjoy it!

41

MITIGATITING SMOOTHIE FREEZER PACK

Fixings

1 cup (5 ounces) solidified mango

1/2 cup (2 ounces) solidified cauliflower florets

1 banana, cut

1" bit of new ginger, stripped

1" piece new turmeric, stripped

squeeze new dark pepper

squeeze cinnamon

1 cup of canned coconut milk

1/2 cup water

1 scoop collagen peptides (discretionary)

To Make Freezer Packs:

Spot all fixings aside from coconut milk and water into a cooler safe sack. Freeze until prepared to use, as long as multi month.

To mix:

Consolidate all fixings, including coconut milk and water in a fast blender.

Mix until velvety, including extra water if important.

42

Grapefruit Detox Smoothie

This grapefruit pineapple detox smoothie is stacked with supplements to help lessen swelling, support your digestion, and make you feel your best!

Fixings

1 Winter Sweets red grapefruit

2 cups solidified pineapple pieces

1/3 cup Greek yogurt

1 Tablespoon coconut oil

1/4 inch handle of new ginger

grapefruit sections, berries, and granola (for topping)

INSTRUCTIONS

Section grapefruit over a bowl so you can gather all the juice. Put 2-3 fragments in a safe spot for fixing. Include grapefruit sections, grapefruit juice, solidified pineapple, Greek yogurt, coconut oil, and new ginger into a powerful blender and mix until smooth. Taste and alter fixings dependent on your inclination. On the off chance that the smoothie is too thick you can include a little non-dairy milk.

Fill two glasses and enjoy it. Or then again serve in a bowl with your preferred fixings — grapefruit fragments, granola, berries, and so on.

43

Velvety Citrus Ginger Smoothie

This Creamy Citrus Ginger Smoothie is the ideal reviving beverage! Made with coconut milk, new ginger, and navel oranges.

INGREDIENTS

2 Navel Oranges, stripped and fragmented

1/2 cup coconut milk (or milk of decision)

1 1" solid shape new ginger, skin evacuated and cleaved

1 cup ice

Guidelines

1. Include the entirety of the fixings into a blender – ensure your oranges are fragmented on the off chance that you incline toward a more mash free squeezed orange.

2. Mix until smooth. Include more ice or fluid for wanted consistency.

44

YAM PIE SMOOTHIE BOWL

Fixings

1 little yam

1/2 cup steamed at that point solidified zucchini*

1 little banana, solidified

1/3 cup yogurt (+ more for garnish)

1/2 cup unsweetened vanilla almond milk (more for a more slender consistency)

1 tsp pumpkin pie zest

1/4 tsp cardamom

new ginger (about the size of your fingernail)

Guidelines

To cook the yam:

cut the yam down the middle and afterward steam in a liner bushel for 10 mins

Or then again enclose by foil and spot in a 350-degree broiler for 60 minutes.

For smoothie:

place all fixings into a blender and mix until smooth.

Top with extra yogurt and pumpkin zest or fixings of decision

It could utilize uncooked zucchini too

45

MANGO ALMOND BUTTER SMOOTHIE

Start your day with this velvety and delightful Mango Almond Butter Smoothie. Made with solidified mango, banana, almond margarine, and milk and protein powder this smoothie will keep you full for quite a long time!

Fixings

1 cup of solidified mango

1/2 solidified banana, cut

1/2 cup almond milk

1 tbsp almond spread

1 scoop vanilla protein powder

discretionary: 2 cups spinach for an additional veggie support.

Directions

Consolidate all fixings in your blender.

Drink right away.

This smoothie is thick so if you like to drink with a straw as opposed to eat with a spoon include more almond milk.

46

Nectar and Wild Blueberry Smoothie

This Honey and Wild Blueberry Smoothie is so straightforward and flavourful. Velvety, reviving, and solid – an incredible, simple breakfast or bite!

1 banana, new or solidified

1 cup mango pieces, new or solidified

1/2 cup wild blueberries, new or solidified

1/2 cup plain non-fat Greek yogurt

1/2 cup milk (or sufficiently only to assist things with mixing easily)

1 stacking tablespoon crude nectar (more to taste)

1/2 cup kale or some other include ins that you need

Directions

Spot bananas, mangoes, blueberries, yogurt, and milk in a blender. Mix until smooth. Include the kale and nectar; mix again until smooth.

Whenever wanted (and particularly if every one of your fixings were new rather than solidified), add a couple of ice 3D shapes to build the volume of the smoothie and assist it with staying chilled. Smash until smooth.

Top with extra blueberries and serve right away.!

47

BLUE SMOOTHIE

Blue Smoothie made with Butterfly Pea Tea Powder. Yummy bananas, nutritious hemp seeds, almond milk, and tea powder is all you requirement for this astounding blue-hued smoothie!

ingredients

2 solidified bananas3 Tbsp hemp seeds

1 cup almond milk (or coconut milk or some other milk of decision)

1-3 tsp Butterfly Pea Tea Powder (contingent upon how blue you need your smoothie)

Instruction - Add all fixings to a rapid blender and afterward serve/

48

WATERMELON SMOOTHIE

World's Best Watermelon Smoothie! Highlighting 4 basic fixings - watermelon, mint, nectar, and water. You are going to go crazy.

Fixings

2 cups solidified cubed watermelon

1 cup of water

1 tablespoon of nectar or different sugars to taste

a couple of mints and additionally basil leaves, in the event that you need to take it to the following level

Guidelines

Mix the watermelon and the water until smooth. Include the nectar and mint and mix another 10-20 seconds until generally smooth and the consistency of a slushy.

Serve right away!

49

Avocado Spinach Smoothie

This Avocado Spinach Smoothie is the creamiest green smoothie you will ever attempt. Besides, the mango gives it an overly sweet tropical taste!

Fixings

1 cup diced solidified mango

1/2 avocado

2 hands full infant spinach

2-3 Tbsp protein powder

1 cup of cold water

Guidelines

Add all fixings to your blender. Mix until smooth. Enjoy right away.

50.

Peach Raspberry Smoothie

This basic smoothie just takes 5 minutes to make and is incredible for breakfast, a sound bite, or even sweet!

Fixings

1 cup cut peaches

1/2 cup solidified raspberries

1 cup vanilla unsweetened almond milk or milk of your decision

1-2 teaspoons agave or nectar relying upon the pleasantness of your peaches

3-4 ice 3D squares

Directions

Add peaches and raspberries to a blender

Include milk, agave or nectar, and ice 3D squares to the blender.

Mix until smooth. Serve right away.

51

Blackberry Lime Smoothie

This straightforward and sound blackberry smoothie is extraordinary for breakfast, nibble time, or even treat! Furthermore, you will never know there is spinach in this smoothie.

Ingredients

1 cup milk or almond milk

6 ounces Original French Vanilla yogurt

1/2 teaspoon lime

Juice of one huge lime

1 cup new spinach

1 cup solidified blackberries

1 solidified banana

Guidelines

Include milk, yogurt, lime pizzazz, lime juice, spinach, blackberries, and banana to the blender. Spot the cover on and mix until smooth. Fill glasses and serve right away.

Continuously keep unpeeled bananas in the frizer for smoothies. On the off chance that you don't have a solidified banana, you can utilize a normal banana and include a couple of ice 3D squares.

52

TROPICAL COCONUT SMOOTHIE BOWL

This tropical coconut smoothie bowl is an empowering breakfast formula made with new products of the soil fixings. The base is loaded up with tropical natural products like mango and pineapple and it is thickened with coconut milk. Top this smoothie bowl with your preferred sound fixings like extra new natural product, chia seeds and granola!

Fixings

2 solidified bananas

1/2 cups solidified pineapple

1 cup of solidified mango

1/2 cup coconut milk shaken

2 tablespoons nectar overlook for the veggie lover alternative

1/4 teaspoon coconut remove

Fixing; mango granola, chia seeds, fruits, other fruit.

INSTRUCTIONS

Include with or without fixings from garnishes in the blender. Mix on high speed for 1-2 minutes until thick and smooth. If you don't have a powerful blender it might take somewhat more.

Fill a huge bowl and include arranged garnishes. Eat right away.

53.

Raspberry Peach Spinach Smoothie

The intriguing thing about brilliant energetic smoothies, for example, this raspberry peach spinach smoothie is the way that the flavours shroud the greens and the shading conceals it as well.

Utilizing organic products that make energetic shaded smoothies is critical on the off chance that you need to deceive your psyche that you are having something healthy

 INGREDIENTS

1 1/3 cup unsweetened almond milk

1/3 cup plain kefir or plain greek yogurt

3 pitted dates

2/3 cup solidified raspberries

3/4 cup solidified peach cuts

A monster bunch of infant spinach leaves

Discretionary ADD-INS

1 tablespoon hemp hearts

1 teaspoon honey bee dust

1 teaspoon maca powder

1-2 tablespoons your preferred nut margarine

Guidelines

Spot all fixings into the blender, with the fluids at the base, at that point mix until smooth and to your ideal consistency. If it is excessively thick, include increasingly fluid. In the event that excessively slim, add some ice to thicken up or progressively solidified organic product.

54

STRAWBERRY BANANA HIDDEN CAULIFLOWER SMOOTHIE

For those out there who are continually attempting to discover approaches to get your little ones to eat vegetables, solidified cauliflower is an incredible method to get them to drink their veggies, particularly in the event that they're not into smoothies made with spinach as a result of the splendid green shading.

Fixings

1 cup solidified cauliflower (ideally riced cauliflower)

1 cup of solidified strawberries

1 solidified banana

1 3/4 cup almond milk

1 tablespoon almond spread

1/2 avocado

2 teaspoons maple syrup or nectar (discretionary)

Bearings

Consolidate all fixings in a powerful blender and mix until smooth.

Fill glasses and trimming with strawberry and banana cuts whenever wanted. Enjoy!

55.

 MOCHA CAULIFLOWER COLD BREW PROTEIN SMOOTHIE

Fixings:

1/2 cup cold blend espresso

1/2 cup unsweetened vanilla almond milk or cashew milk (+ a sprinkle of entire milk)

3/4 cup solidified crude cauliflower

1/2 scoop chocolate protein powder

1 tablespoon collagen

1 tablespoon cocoa powder

Bearings:

Spot everything into a high-powered blender and mix until smooth.

Fill a cup and appreciate!

56

HELPEED UP DAIRY-FREE ORANGE SMOOTHIE

This san dairy orange smoothie is pressed with a

fruity flavour and made with new orange pizzazz, vanilla, ice 3D shapes, rich coconut milk, and unsweetened vanilla almond milk.

Fixings

6 solidified ice blocks (around 3/4 cup)

1/2 cup full-fat coconut milk

1/3 cup unsweetened vanilla almond milk

1 orange, stripped (with any seeds expelled) + pizzazz

Sprinkle of vanilla concentrate

Guidelines

Spot all fixings into a high-powdered blender.

Mix and appreciate!

57

Green Monster Smoothie

An extraordinary approach to sneak greens into your smoothie - and you cannot taste it. This green beast smoothie is an incredible method to sneak a few greens into your day.

Fixings

2 cups solidified organic product (I utilized blended natural product that included pineapples grapes, strawberries, mangos, and peaches)

1 banana broken into pieces

1/2 cup almond milk

Enormous bunch of spinach

Guidelines

Toss everything in the blender and mix until a smooth consistency. If it stalls out, turn it off, and go through a spatula to break it and start it once more.

58

Peachy Green Smoothie

Sneak those veggies into this smoothie and your children will NEVER know!

INGREDIENTS

2 cups coconut milk refreshment, NOT the canned coconut milk

2 cups solidified cut peaches

2 solidified underripe bananas, cut

1 teaspoon ground new ginger, discretionary

2 cups inexactly pressed spinach leaves

Guidelines

Empty the coconut milk into a blender and include the peaches, banana, ginger (on the off chance that utilizing), at that point the spinach.

Mix until smooth.

59

Blended Berry Smoothie Bowl

This blended berry smoothie bowl is a fun better approach to "drink" a smoothie while including your most loved toppings!

INGREDIENTS

1 cup coconut milk drink, not from the can

2/3 cup solidified blended berries

1 huge banana

2 tablespoons cashew spread, or your preferred nut margarine

Your preferred garnishes: natural product, granola, chia seeds, and so forth.

Guidelines

Empty the coconut milk into the base of the blender container. At that point include the solidified berries, banana, and cashew spread on top. Safely place the cover on the container and mix until no pieces remain. You may need to stop and mix it around if it is excessively thick.

Empty smoothie into a bowl and spot garnishes on top.

60

GINGER SMOOTHIE

Ginger enables the body to benefit as much as possible from these supplements by considering legitimate supplement assimilation. This implies ginger advances a sound stomach related framework by ensuring that nothing gets supported up and everything is put to acceptable use.

INGREDIENTS

1 cup spinach (new)

1 cup almond milk (unsweetened)

1/2 banana

1 apple (any assortment, center evacuated)

1/4 inch ginger (stripped)

Directions

Mix spinach and almond milk together until smooth.

Include remaining fixings and mix once more.

NOTES

Use at any rate one solidified organic product to make the smoothie cold

Notwithstanding controlling digestion, ginger additionally advances a solid insusceptible framework since it assists clean with trip microscopic organisms in the colon. Pair this with all the supplements found in apples and you can be certain that you are benefiting as much as possible from the supplements accessible in your Ginger Smoothie

Pairings For A Better Weight-Loss Smoothies

The standard of combining healthy recipes to make a more effective healthy combo applies to what you decide to place in your weight loss smoothies every morning.

 It could not be any more obvious, a few fixings work best à deux by boosting every others' supplement retention or improving taste or surface.

There are sure nourishments that have synergistic associations with another, So in spite of the fact that the nourishments might be amazing all alone—think superfoods like kale and berries—they might be much more grounded as a piece of a couple.

 In view of that, we went to nourishment specialists to get a couple of their preferred powerful pairs. Here, the fixing sets that help your smoothie help you.

1. Green Tea + Kiwi

Lunch time is not only an evening movement and tea doesn't need to be tasted alone. As opposed to utilize overwhelming milk or yogurt for the base of your smoothie, blend things up for summer and select green tea.

 Nourishments that are plentiful in nutrient C like kiwi (it has a higher grouping of the supplement than an orange) help support the retention of catechins from green tea—cell reinforcements that assist fry with fatting and transform it into vitality. You will require that for the steamier months!

2 Blueberries + Cottage Cheese

This couple hits you with a one-two punch of cell reinforcements and lean protein and, to sweeten the deal even further, the curds thickens the smoothie to a nearly milkshake-like consistency. Breakfast or pastry, this smoothie gets the green light.

3 Tofu + Blackberries

The nutrient D in tofu will help support ingestion of bone-sound calcium from the blackberries. Additionally, like curds, tofu thickens up your smoothie and furthermore helps counter a portion of the poignancy from the blackberries.

The regular protein substance of the smoothie will likewise permit you to dump paunch swelling whey powders.

4 Strawberries + Kale

Without a doubt, kale is a superfood, yet that does not mean it's extraordinary at everything. It needs a sidekick! The nutrient C in strawberries improves the ingestion of kale's iron substance—and this could be especially significant for any veggie lovers that may not be getting enough of the supplement.

5 Avocados + Spinach

Carrots are not the main eye defenders; trade your titbit time veg for at the beginning of today smoothie for similar advantages without all the eating. This team will give you a lift before you even get the chance to work. The solid fat in avocados improves the cancer prevention agent lutein in spinach to support eye wellbeing—it might guard you from age-related macular degeneration and waterfalls—the two of which may prompt debilitated vision and visual impairment.

6 Almonds + Banana

Solidified bananas are the best mystery of the smoothie world; they give your smoothie a milkshake-like consistency that is ideal for banishing those difficult sweet tooth-actuated yearnings.

Add a few almonds to keep your vitality level high well until noon; the fibre and protein in these nuts assistance hinder the retention of characteristic sugar from bananas, keeping blood glucose levels increasingly steady.

7. Pecans + Baby Spinach

If this seems like an improbable matching to you, simply envision them mixed up with a solidified banana, some nutty spread, and a sprinkle of almond milk.

 You will not taste the verdant greens. Omega-3 unsaturated fats in pecans help support the retention of nutrient K found in spinach. Nutrient K is a triple danger that assists with cell development, blood flow, and keeps the bones solid.

8 Pecans + Pumpkin

The unsaturated fat found in walnuts assists with the ingestion of the pumpkin's nutrient A substance, which underpins the skin, invulnerable framework, and mucous layers.

Only three ounces of canned pumpkin gives triple the day by day estimation of the nutrient. Include some cinnamon or pumpkin pie flavour for a sweet roused start to the day.

9 Cayenne + Cocoa Powder

If you are new to this combo, do not discount it currently. Cayenne upgrades the pleasantness of the cocoa, and its flavonoids fill in as cancer prevention agents that help battle irritation. What is more, investigate proposes that capsaicin, a functioning fixing in cayenne, may assist lowering blood pressure, battle fat and smother craving.

In addition, it might likewise somewhat help digestion. Mix them along with a solidified cut banana and some almond milk for a morning meal smoothie that poses a flavour like solidified hot cocoa.

10 Tangerines + Soft Tofu

Cause your smoothie to mirror the changing season by utilizing citrus as your essential organic product. The ascorbic corrosive, an invulnerable framework defender, in tangerines enables the body to retain iron from tofu.

The light stuff contains 40 percent of the day by day needs of the supplement, so think of it as a moderately strong source. For a youth treat-propelled drink, mixed it with some vanilla plant-protein powder. The tangerine and vanilla consolidate to make an adult form of a Creamsicle.

11. Hemp Seeds + Coconut Oil

The medium-chain triglycerides found in coconut oil may help increment magnesium retention from hemp seeds. This mineral not just assists with rest issues and bone thickness yet additionally cuts atherosclerosis and hypertension chance.

Try not to give the fat access coconut oil frighten you away. This sound fat gives your smoothies a liberal surface as well as helps shave your centre.

12 Avocado + Papaya

Cannot escape this year? Channel the tropics with this thinning and fulfilling morning smoothie. The monounsaturated fat in avocados assists with fat-solvent (and vision-securing, cell development supporting) nutrient A ingestion from papaya—a natural product that likewise happens to contain double the day by day proposal.

13 Almond Butter + Kale

Kale may add shading to your smoothie, yet on the off chance that you mix up the correct fixings, you will not taste the green option. Join almond spread, almond milk, a cut solidified banana, cocoa powder, and a bunch of kale for a nutty spread cup-propelled smoothie. Kale contains a heavy portion of both nutrient A and nutrient K—206 percent of the day by day estimation of the previous and 684 percent of the everyday estimation of the last mentioned—and the monounsaturated fats in almond spread assistance support ingestion of these two supplements.

Approaches to Supercharge Your Smoothie For Weight Loss

Smoothies can quick track supplements into your body and top you off in simply an issue of tastes. By picking supplement thick, protein-stuffed, fibre-rich, and low-calorie fixings, you'll have the option to invigorate your body with the fuel it needs to consume fat, form muscle and control wacky longings.

With the correct fixings, your morning meal smoothies can stir up your whole weight reduction plan—and in the most ideal way possible! Smoothies can quick track supplements into your body and top you off in simply a question of tastes.

By deciding on supplement thick, protein-pressed, fibre-rich, you'll have the option to strengthen your body with the fuel it needs to consume fat, form muscle and control wacky yearnings

In this way, dust off your blender, avoid the neighbourhood smoothie joint, and begin preparing your own gut busting drinks by adding these powerhouse fixings to your shopping list.

Furthermore, to lose considerably more weight—as much as 16 pounds in 14 days

1   Maca

Local to Peru, Maca has been touted as a superfood credited with improving vitality, endurance, memory, and richness. While maca is not sans calorie, it could be your pass to progressively proficient exercises. "I would suggest beginning with about portion of a teaspoon and work up to about a tablespoon.

Individuals find that it gives them a pleasant buzz without having any caffeine content. The more vitality you have and the more you last at the exercise centre, the more calories you are going to consume by and large.

2   Matcha

Vitality levels direct something beyond your state of mind, they additionally intensely impact your food decisions for the duration of the day and your capacity to really make it to the exercise centre.

There is more caffeine in it than customary green tea since it's the entire leaf ground up, but at the same time it's an incredible wellspring of cancer prevention agents and is for all intents and purposes sans calorie. The match is additionally exceptionally special as a result of its weight reduction superpowers.

3   Pumpkin

You do not need to trust that Fall will receive the midsection shaving rewards of this super squash. Pumpkin contains some fibre and is a decent wellspring of beta-carotene and potassium, which is an electrolyte [important for legitimate muscle function]. Recall that pumpkin is certifiably not a 'free food", however you can consider it making up half of your natural product parcel in your smoothie. Stick with unsweetened canned pumpkin and mix with 33% of a banana first. From that point take a stab at including things like cinnamon and Greek yogurt for a delicious, filling, and diet-accommodating shake.

4   Flaxseed

These unassuming seeds brag high measures of omega-3 unsaturated fats are a rich wellspring of cell reinforcements called lignans, and furthermore present a decent portion of fibre. Additionally? A Harvard University study connected the utilization of flaxseed to a 37 percent expansion in weight reduction. Keep a pack of ground flaxseed in your ice chest and add a spoonful to shakes to help dissolve away the pounds. Why ground? Since you get more nourishment from them that way.

5   Chia Seeds

At the point when you need to get more fit it would profit you significantly to go to fibre-rich nourishments since they top you off and help murder off low quality nourishment yearnings.

These little seeds pack a robust 11 grams in an interesting two tablespoons. Chia is likewise what is known as a hydrophilic food, which implies they absorb water—and a great deal of it, as well! Chia seeds extend to multiple times their size when risen in fluid, so adding them to your shake will keep your paunch full, your craving crushed, and your outline smooth.

6	Clean Protein Powder
Enhancing with clean protein powder, liberated from any counterfeit added substances is a decent method to siphon up the totality factor of your shake—simply be careful about the amount you are utilizing.
Smoothies can be a wonderful method to get supplements, however, they can likewise be an overwhelming hitter for calories. It is particularly imperative to see how to arrange a smoothie out. I propose that you adhere to similar standards and guidelines that you do when you are making it at home.
 So, when you head to the juice bar for your post-exercise recuperation shake, do not be hesitant to request to see the compartment the protein comes in or to get some information about explicit extents.

7	Vegan Protein Powder

Continuously remember one protein or one solid fat for your smoothies. For protein attempt a plant-based protein powder or a spotless whey protein—Greek yogurt checks, too. Not exclusively will protein add to satiety, yet it will likewise aid muscle development and fix and support more prominent calorie consuming, therefore. Plant-based protein powders are a decent choice on the off chance that you have an increasingly touchy stomach.

8   Cinnamon

Some superfoods can be calorie-loaded, and some can contain none by any stretch of the imagination, [so be aware of what and the amount you are including in]. A portion of my preferred sans calorie decisions are things like cinnamon or turmeric—the two of which are calming and contain cell reinforcements that are sound for you. Cinnamon helps support the flavour and dietary profile of your smoothie, with no additional calories or sugar, making it simple for you to remain on target with your eating regimen.

9   Oats

You might be accustomed to spooning oats in your mouth for breakfast, however, begin making this fibre-rich staple a customary in your mixing schedule. No compelling reason to concoct them—dump folded oats straight into your blender with the remainder of your elements for a thick shake that will keep you full and vitality consistent gratitude to the fibre found in oats.

10   Turmeric

Turmeric is the dynamic fixing in curry yet it is for all intents and purposes flavourless, so you can blend it in with anything. It is incredible for your joints and can help direct glucose. At the point when your glucose is steady you won't experience exceptional highs and lows in vitality, and thus, will make more advantageous more midriff well-disposed food decisions, so don't avoid this splendidly toned flavour.

11   Nut Butter

Regardless of whether you feel weak at the knees over almond, nut, pecan or cashew margarine, it does not make a difference, they all offer an increase in sound omega-3 unsaturated fats.

As indicated by an investigation from the University of South Australia, an eating routine wealthy in omega-3 fats joined with customary exercise can assist you with losing more weight than simply practice alone. Simply do not go over the edge with your scoops. A limit of two tablespoons of nuts or nut margarine in your beverages since they are viewed as a calorie-thick food.

12   Almond Milk

At this point it ought to be evident that on the off chance that you need to free yourself of undesirable pounds you must free your eating routine of superfluous sugar and calories, and with regards to smoothies utilizing juice as a fluid base is a major no-no.

 That is the reason it is ideal to adhere to fluids like water or low-sugar almond milk when mixing. You need to purchase unsweetened almond or coconut milk, and furthermore remember that on the off chance that you make your own almond milk the calories will be higher in light of the fact that the procedure is not quite the same as how they make it.

13   Spinach

At the point when you're searching for straightforward approaches to shed pounds, you can never have an excessive number of veggies— they're low in calories and high in supplements that help your body work at its most elevated level. Continuously attempt to add a vegetable or two to smoothies. There is no restriction on what number of veggies you can place in. Spinach is a standout amongst other green choices for smoothies since its flavour is less articulated than different veggies, and it additionally mixes up pleasantly in shakes, so you won't taste any green pieces through your straw.

14   Ginger

Ginger might be a definitive disturbed stomach cure, however because of its calming powers it additionally can upgrade your weight reduction endeavours.
Including new ginger into smoothies not exclusively will give your beverage a kick and mask any harsh greens, yet it will enable your body to process the nourishments you are swallowing down.

 By supporting assimilation, ginger enables your body to retain more supplements and puts forth your solid attempts progressively charming by and large. It's additionally a low-calorie approach to truly upgrade the flavour of your beverage and is particularly decent when matched with lemon juice.

15   Frozen Banana

Bananas are a smoothie backbone, yet solidified bananas explicitly can take your smoothie game to the next level. At the point when mixed solidified, bananas transform your shake into an overly smooth and thick liberal shake—and when something tastes incredible, you are bound to keep eating it. Simply make certain to adhere to one banana or less to stay quiet about calories and sugar.

16   Avocado

Avocado is an especially extraordinary wellspring of monounsaturated fats; study shows that an eating regimen wealthy in these sorts of fats may really assist spot with decreasing stomach fat by controlling the declaration of certain fat qualities. Adhering to 33% of avocado in shakes to monitor calories while yet getting those filling supplements is perfect.

17   Water

It might appear disappointing, however utilizing water as your fluid base in smoothies can assist you with eliminating genuine calories and sugar instead of well-known squeezes or milk. It will likewise kick up the hydration factor of your mix, as well.

Try not to stress over a watered-down flavour either, provided that you're including all the great stuff—organic products, veggies, and rich nut margarine—you won't notice the replacement.

18   Greek Yogurt

On the off chance that you are not one for powdered protein, at that point go to this rich, protein-stuffed, probiotic powerhouse to get your fill of the supplement. Those following a low-calorie diet more extravagant in protein increased more muscle and lost more fat than those devouring a low-calorie diet low in protein. Because of its velvety, thick surface, Greek yogurt will likewise change your shakes into a greater amount of a guilty pleasure.

19   Goji

Well known in conventional Chinese medication because of its high cell reinforcement content, goji berries have discovered their way into current kitchens of the wellbeing cognizant. Despite the fact that they've been touted as an invulnerability supporter and as a sort of "wellspring of youth" for maturing skin, goji berries are an ideal smoothie include in light of the fact that they are lower in sugar and a decent wellspring of fibre.

 Spring for goji powder or absorb the berries in water first, at that point mix. The tang will fulfil your sweet tooth and the fibre will help top you off and keep you customary. Devouring goji berry squeeze routinely can expand general sentiments of prosperity and bliss.

20   Acai

Acai is another most loved superfood among the smooth and weight-cognizant in light of the fact that it's normally lower in sugar than different foods grown from the ground a taste that is suggestive of red wine blended in with notes of chocolate. Acai can without much of a stretch be found in the solidified segment sold in little divided out bundles, which are anything but difficult to tear open and hurl in the blender.

 Acai is effortlessly consumed by the body when devoured as a juice or mash, which implies that you will adequately hold a greater amount of the supplements from the cancer prevention agent rich natural product.

21   Raw Cocoa Powder

Chocolate may really assist you with getting more fit—truly, help you! — and there's exploration to demonstrate it. Negligibly prepared cocoa is low in sugar and stacked with cancer prevention agents and study shows that the flavanols in chocolate may help diminish muscle to fat ratio. While picking a crude cocoa powder you need to take a gander at the mark and check how handled it is. The more handled it is, the more fixings it will have. It will say crude on the off chance that it has not been warmed, which is the thing that you need so you get more advantages from the cocoa bean.

22   Coconut Oil

Bringing oils into your eating regimen can be precarious in light of the fact that not all are made equivalent nor are they using any and all means low in calories, in any case, it would profit your midriff to keep coconut oil supplied consistently.

Utilizing a teaspoon of coconut oil in smoothies is somewhat sweet and not overly solid, and there is some genuinely acceptable, inquire about on coconut oil being advantageous to thyroid wellbeing in modest quantities.

It additionally considers a fat, so it can assist keep with blooding sugar more consistent. A sound thyroid and consistent glucose can both help incredibly in weight reduction endeavours.

The 20 Most Weight-Loss-Friendly Foods

Not all calories are made equivalent. Various nourishments experience diverse metabolic pathways in our bodies.

They can have unfathomably various impacts on your yearning, hormones, and the quantity of calories you consume.

Here are the 20 most weight reduction amicable nourishments on earth that are bolstered by science.

1. Entire Eggs

Once dreaded for being high in cholesterol, entire eggs have been making a rebound.

Albeit a high admission of eggs raises the degrees of "awful" LDL-cholesterol in certain individuals, they are probably the best food to eat on the off chance that you have to get more fit. They are high in protein and fat and are very satisfying.

One investigation in 30 overweight ladies indicated that having eggs for breakfast, rather than bagels, expanded sentiments of totality (satiety) and caused members to eat less for the following 36 hours.

An additional eight-week study found that eggs for breakfast expanded weight reduction on a calorie-limited eating regimen, contrasted with bagels.

Eggs are likewise unimaginably supplement thick and can assist you with getting all the supplements you need on a calorie-confined eating routine. Strangely, practically all the supplements are found in the yolks.

2. Verdant Greens

Verdant greens incorporate kale, spinach, collards, swiss chards, and a couple of others. They have a few properties that make them ideal for a weight reduction diet, for example, being low in calories and starches and stacked with fiber. Eating verdant greens is an extraordinary method to expand the volume of your dinners, without expanding the calories. Various examinations show that dinners and diets with low vitality thickness cause individuals to eat less calories generally speaking.

Verdant greens are additionally fantastically nutritious and high in numerous nutrients, cancer prevention agents and minerals, including calcium, which has been appeared to help fat consuming.

Verdant greens are an astounding expansion to your weight reduction diet. In addition to the fact that they are low in calories high in fiber that helps keep you feeling full.

3. Salmon

Greasy fish like salmon is unbelievably sound and fulfilling, keeping you full for a long time with moderately barely any calories. Salmon is stacked with top notch protein, sound fats and different significant supplements.

Fish — and fish when all is said in done — may likewise flexibly a lot of iodine.

This supplement is essential for legitimate thyroid capacity, which is critical to keep your digestion running ideally.

Studies show that countless individuals don't fill their iodine needs.

Salmon is additionally stacked with omega-3 unsaturated fats, which have been appeared to help decrease aggravation, which is known to assume a significant job in corpulence and metabolic disease settling on it a decent decision for a solid weight reduction diet

Mackerel, trout, sardines, herring and different kinds of greasy fish are likewise phenomenal.

4. Cruciferous Vegetables

Cruciferous vegetables incorporate broccoli, cauliflower, cabbage, and Brussels grows. Like different vegetables, they're high in fiber and will in general be extraordinarily filling.

Likewise, these kinds of veggies for the most part contain not too bad measures of protein.

They're not close to as high in protein as creature nourishments or vegetables yet at the same time high contrasted with most vegetables.

A blend of protein, fiber and low vitality thickness makes cruciferous vegetables the ideal nourishments to remember for your dinners in the event that you have to get thinner.

They're likewise profoundly nutritious and contain malignant growth battling substances

They are low in calories however high in fiber and supplements. Adding them to your eating routine isn't just a magnificent weight reduction system yet may likewise improve your general wellbeing.

5. Lean Beef and Chicken Breast

Meat has been unjustifiably slandered.

It has been accused for different medical issues in spite of an absence of good proof to back up these negative cases.

Despite the fact that prepared meat is undesirable, examines show that natural red meat doesn't raise the danger of coronary illness or diabetes.

Truly, meat is a weight reduction agreeable food since it's high in protein.

Protein is by a long shot the most filling supplement, and eating a high-protein diet can cause you to wreck to 80–100 additional calories for each day.

Studies have indicated that expanding your protein admission to 25–% of every day calories can cut longings by 60%, diminish your craving for late-evening eating significantly and cause weight reduction of right around one pound (0.45 kg) every week

In case you're on a low-carb diet, don't hesitate to eat greasy meats. Be that as it may, in case you're on a moderate-to a high-sugar diet, picking lean meats might be progressively suitable.

Eating natural lean meat is a superb method to expand your protein admission. Supplanting a portion of the carbs or fat in your eating routine with protein could make it simpler for you to lose overabundance fat.

6. Bubbled Potatoes

White potatoes appear to have become undesirable for reasons unknown.

Notwithstanding, they have a few properties that make them an ideal food — both for weight reduction and ideal wellbeing.

They contain a fantastically assorted scope of supplements — a tad of nearly all that you need.

There have even been records of individuals living on only potatoes alone for broadened timeframes.

They're especially high in potassium, a supplement that a great many people don't get enough of and that assumes a significant job in circulatory strain control.

On a scale called the Satiety Index, which gauges how filling various nourishments are, white, bubbled potatoes scored the most elevated of the considerable number of food sources tried.

This means by eating white, bubbled potatoes, you will normally feel full and eat less of different nourishments.

On the off chance that you permit potatoes to cool for some time in the wake of bubbling, they will shape high measures of safe starch, a fiber-like substance that has been appeared to have different medical advantages, including weight reduction.

Yams, turnips, and other root vegetables are additionally fantastic.

Bubbled potatoes are among the most filling nourishments. They're especially acceptable at decreasing your hunger, possibly smothering your food consumption later in the day.

7. Fish

Fish is another low-calorie, high-protein food. It's lean fish, which means it's low in fat.

Fish is well known among weight lifters and wellness models who're on a cut, as it's an extraordinary method to expand protein consumption while keeping complete calories and fat low.

In case you're attempting to underscore protein consumption, try to pick fish canned in water, not oil.

Fish is a fantastic, lean wellspring of top notch protein. Supplanting different macronutrients, for example, carbs or fat, with protein is a successful weight reduction technique on a calorie-limited eating regimen.

8. Beans and Legumes

A few beans and different vegetables can be gainful for weight reduction. This incorporates lentils, dark beans, kidney beans, and some others.

These nourishments will in general be high in protein and fiber, which are two supplements that have been appeared to prompt satiety.

They additionally will in general contain some safe starch.

The primary issue is that many individuals experience issues enduring vegetables. Therefore, it's imperative to set them up appropriately.

Beans and vegetables are a decent expansion to your weight reduction diet. They're both high in protein and fiber, adding to sentiments of totality and lower calorie admission.

9. Soups

As referenced above, dinners and diets with low vitality thickness will in general cause individuals to eat less calories.

Most nourishments with a low vitality thickness are those that contain bunches of water, for example, vegetables and natural products.

Yet, you can likewise simply add water to your food, making a soup.

A few examinations have indicated that eating precisely the same food transformed into a soup as opposed to as strong food, causes individuals to feel progressively satisfied and eat fundamentally less calories/

Simply make a point not to add an excessive amount of fat to your soup, for example, cream or coconut milk, as this can fundamentally expand its calorie content.

Soups can be a successful piece of a weight reduction diet. Their high water content makes them very filling. Be that as it may, attempt to maintain a strategic distance from rich or slick soups.

10. Curds

Dairy items will in general be high in protein.

Perhaps the best one is curds, which — calorie for calorie — is for the most part protein with not very many carbs and minimal fat.

Eating curds is an incredible method to help your protein consumption. It's likewise very satisfying, causing you to feel full with a moderately low number of calories.

Dairy items are additionally high in calcium, which may help fat consuming

Other low-fat, high-protein dairy items incorporate Greek yogurt and skyr.

Eating lean dairy items, for example, curds, is probably the most ideal approaches to get more protein without essentially expanding your calorie admission.

11. Avocados

Avocados are a one of a kind organic product. While most organic products are high in carbs, avocados are stacked with sound fats.

They're especially high in monounsaturated oleic corrosive, a similar kind of fat found in olive oil.

In spite of being for the most part fat, avocados likewise contain a great deal of water and fiber, making them less vitality thick than you may might suspect.

Furthermore, they're an ideal expansion to vegetable servings of mixed greens, as studies show that their fat substance can build carotenoid cancer prevention agent retention from the vegetables 2.6-to 15-crease.

They additionally contain numerous significant supplements, including fiber and potassium.

Avocados are a genuine case of a sound fat source you can remember for your eating regimen while attempting to get thinner. Simply make a point to keep your admission moderate.

12. Apple Cider Vinegar

Apple juice vinegar is staggeringly well known in the characteristic wellbeing network. It's regularly utilized in fixings like dressings or vinaigrettes, and a few people even weaken it in water and drink it.

A few human-based examinations recommend that apple juice vinegar can be helpful for weight reduction.

Taking vinegar simultaneously as a high-carb supper can expand sentiments of completion and cause individuals to eat 200–275 fewer calories for the remainder of the day.
One 12-week study in obese individuals also showed that 15 or 30 ml of vinegar per day caused a weight loss of 2.6–3.7 pounds, or 1.2–1.7 kilograms.

Vinegar has also been shown to reduce blood sugar spikes after meals, which may have various beneficial health effects in the long term.

Adding apple cider vinegar to your vegetable salad may help curb your appetite, potentially leading to greater weight loss.

13. Nuts
Despite being high in fat, nuts are not as fattening
as you would expect.

They're an excellent snack, containing balanced
amounts of protein, fiber, and healthy fats.

Studies have shown that eating nuts can improve
metabolic health and even promote weight loss.

What's more, population studies have shown that
people who eat nuts tend to be healthier and leaner
than those who don't.

Just make sure not to go overboard, as they're still
fairly high in calories. If you tend to binge and eat
massive amounts of nuts, it may be best to avoid
them.

Nuts can make a healthy addition to an effective
weight loss diet when consumed in moderation.

14. Whole Grains
Though cereal grains have received a bad reputation
in recent years, some types are definitely healthy.

This includes some whole grains that are loaded
with fiber and contain a decent amount of protein.

Notable examples include oats, brown rice, and
quinoa.

Oats are loaded with beta-glucans, soluble fibers that have been shown to increase satiety and improve metabolic health.

Both brown and white rice can contain significant amounts of resistant starch, particularly if cooked and then allowed to cool afterward.

Keep in mind that refined grains are not a healthy choice, and sometimes foods that have "whole grains" on the label are highly processed junk foods that are both harmful and fattening.

If you're on a very low-carb diet, you'll want to avoid grains, as they're high in carbs.

But there's otherwise nothing wrong with eating whole grains if you can tolerate them.

You should avoid refined grains if you're trying to lose weight. Choose whole grains instead — they're much higher in fiber and other nutrients.

15. Chili Pepper
Eating chili peppers may be useful on a weight loss diet.

They contain capsaicin, a substance that has been shown to reduce appetite and increase fat burning in some studies.

This substance is even sold in supplement form and a common ingredient in many commercial weight loss supplements.

One study showed that eating 1 gram of red chili pepper reduced appetite and increased fat burning in people who didn't regularly eat peppers.

However, there was no effect in people who were accustomed to eating spicy food, indicating that a certain level of tolerance can build up.
Eating spicy foods that contain chili peppers may reduce your appetite temporarily and even increase fat burning. However, tolerance seems to build up in those who eat chili regularly.

16. Fruit
Most health experts agree that fruit is healthy.

Numerous population studies have shown that people who eat the most fruit (and vegetables) tend to be healthier than people who don't.
Of course, correlation does not equal causation, so these studies don't prove anything. However, fruits do have properties that make them weight-loss-friendly.

Even though they contain natural sugar, they have a low energy density and take a while to chew. Plus, their fiber content helps prevent sugar from being released too quickly into your bloodstream.

The only people who may want to avoid or minimize fruit are those on a very low-carb, ketogenic diet or have an intolerance.

For most fruits can be an effective and delicious addition to a weight loss diet.

Though fruits contain some sugar, you can easily include them on a weight loss diet. They're high in fiber, antioxidants, and various nutrients that slow the rise of blood sugar after meals.

17. Grapefruit
One fruit that deserves to be highlighted is grapefruit. Its effects on weight control have been studied directly.

In a 12-week study in 91 obese individuals, eating half a fresh grapefruit before meals led to weight loss of 3.5 pounds (1.6 kg).

The grapefruit group also had reduced insulin resistance, a metabolic abnormality that is implicated in various chronic diseases.

Therefore, eating half a grapefruit about half an hour before some of your daily meals may help you feel more satiated and eat fewer overall calories.

Studies indicate that grapefruit may suppress appetite and reduce calorie intake when eaten before meals. It's worth a try if you're want to lose weight.

18. Chia Seeds
Chia seeds are among the most nutritious foods on
the planet.
They contain 12 grams of carbohydrates per ounce
(28 grams), which is pretty high, but 11 of these
grams are fiber.

This makes chia seeds low-carb-friendly food and
one of the best sources of fiber in the world.

Because of its high fiber content, chia seeds can
absorb up to 11–12 times their weight in water,
turning gel-like and expanding in your stomach.

Though some studies have shown that chia seeds
can help reduce appetite, they did not find a
statistically significant effect on weight loss.

However, given their nutrient composition, it makes
sense that chia seeds could be a useful part of your
weight loss diet.

Chia seeds are very high in fiber, which fills you up
and reduces appetite. For this reason, they can be
useful on a weight loss diet.

19. Coconut Oil
Not all fats are created equal. Coconut oil is high in
fatty acids of a medium length, called medium-
chain triglycerides (MCTs).

These fatty acids have been shown to boost satiety
better than other fats and increase the number of
calories burned.
What's more, two studies — one in women and the
other in men — showed that coconut oil reduced
amounts of belly fat.
Of course, coconut oil still contains calories, so
adding it on top of what you're already eating is a
bad idea.

It's not about adding coconut oil to your diet but
about replacing some of your other cooking fats
with coconut oil.

However, studies show that coconut oil is less
satiating than MCT oil — a supplement that
contains much higher numbers of medium-chain
triglycerides.

Extra virgin olive oil is worth mentioning here, as
it's probably one of the healthiest fats on the planet.
Coconut oil contains medium-chain triglycerides
(MCTs) that may increase satiety after meals. MCT
oil supplements are even more effective.

20. Full-Fat Yogurt
Yogurt is another excellent dairy food.

Certain types of yogurt contain probiotic bacteria
that can improve the function of your gut.

Having a healthy gut may help protect against inflammation and leptin resistance, which is one of the main hormonal drivers of obesity.

Make sure to choose yogurt with live, active cultures, as other types of yogurt contain virtually no probiotics.

Also, consider choosing full-fat yogurt. Studies show that full-fat dairy — but not low-fat — is associated with a reduced risk of obesity and type 2 diabetes over time.

Low-fat yogurt is usually loaded with sugar, so it's best to avoid it.
Probiotic yogurt can increase your digestive health. Consider adding it to your weight loss diet but make sure to avoid products that contain added sugar.

The Bottom Line
It's easy to find healthy foods to include on a weight loss diet.

These are mainly whole foods like fish, lean meat, vegetables, fruit, nuts, seeds, and legumes.

Several processed foods, such as probiotic yogurt, extra-virgin olive oil, and oatmeal are also excellent choices.

Along with moderation and regular exercise, eating these nutritious foods should pave your way to success and healthier life.